WITHDRAWN
WRIGHT STATE UNIVERSITY LIBRARIES

OXFORD MEDICAL PUBLICATIONS

The Nature of Alcohol and Drug Related Problems

The Nature of Alcohol and Drug Related Problems

SOCIETY FOR THE STUDY OF ADDICTION
MONOGRAPH NO. 2

Edited by

MALCOLM LADER
Professor of Clinical Psychopharmacology
National Addiction Centre
Institute of Psychiatry
University of London

GRIFFITH EDWARDS
Professor of Addiction Behaviour
National Addiction Centre
Institute of Psychiatry
University of London

and

D. COLIN DRUMMOND
Lecturer in Addiction Behaviour
National Addiction Centre
Institute of Psychiatry
University of London

Oxford   New York   Tokyo
OXFORD UNIVERSITY PRESS
1992

Oxford University Press, Walton Street, Oxford OX2 6DP
Oxford   New York   Toronto
Delhi   Bombay   Calcutta   Madras   Karachi
Petaling Jaya   Singapore   Hong Kong   Tokyo
Nairobi   Dar es Salaam   Cape Town
Melbourne   Auckland
and associated companies in
Berlin   Ibadan

Oxford is a trade mark of Oxford University Press

Published in the United States
by Oxford University Press, New York

© Society for the Study of Addiction, 1992

All rights reserved. No part of this publication may be reproduced, stored in a retrieval system, or transmitted, in any form or by any means, electronic, mechanical, photocopying, recording, or otherwise, without the prior permission of Oxford University Press

A catalogue record for this book is available from the British Library

Library of Congress Cataloging-in-Publication Data
The Nature of alcohol and drug related problems / edited by Malcolm Lader, Griffith Edwards, D. Colin Drummond.
p.   cm. — (Oxford medical publications) (Monograph / Society for the Study of Addiction; no. 2)
Consists mostly of papers presented at a meeting in April 1990 at Cumberland Lodge, in Windsor Great Park, Berkshire, U.K.
Includes index.
1. Substance abuse — Congresses. 2. Alcoholism — Congresses.
I. Lader, Malcolm Harold. II. Edwards, Griffith. III. Drummond, D. Colin. IV. Series. V. Series: Monograph (Society for the Study of Addiction); no. 2.
[DNLM: 1. Substance Abuse — congresses. 2. Substance Dependence — congresses. W1 MO5558L no. 2 / WM 270 N287775 1990]
RC563.2.N36   1992   616.86 — dc20   91-39676
ISBN 0 19 262138 6

Typeset by
Graphicraft Typesetters Ltd., Hong Kong
Printed and bound in Great Britain by
Bookcraft (Bath) Ltd., Midsomer Norton, Avon

Preface

The Society for the Study of Addiction was originally founded in 1884 as the Society for the Study and Cure of Inebriety. It held annual meetings and, from the start, published a journal which, after a few changes of title, is now published monthly as the *British Journal of Addiction*. It is now acknowledged as the leading journal in its field.

The Society has broadened its interests to include all substances of abuse. Its membership is now over 500, and covers a very wide range of expertise and background. It holds very successful annual meetings that focus on a theme, but also include communications from the membership.

To complement these open meetings it was decided to hold a small meeting every two years for invited participants, world experts in their field, who would debate, informally, a topic of fundamental interest and concern to those working in the area of substance abuse. The first subject chosen was 'The Nature of Drug Dependence'. The proceedings of this meeting were published in 1990 as the first monograph in the series for the Society for the Study of Addiction.

The second meeting took as its theme, 'Substance Misuse — What Makes "Problems"?' A carefully selected group of participants from a very wide range of disciplines were invited to the discussions, held in April 1990 at Cumberland Lodge, in Windsor Great Park, Berkshire, UK, a venue of great historical interest and architectural beauty set in bucolic surroundings. The format was for the papers to be pre-circulated so that each invited speaker had only to introduce his theme briefly before opening up the discussion. A Hansard short-hand writer provided a verbatim account of the discussions which were later edited.

This book includes the original papers presented at the meeting and edited transcripts of discussions. Additional material has also been commissioned by the Society in order to expand the range of topics covered, beyond that of the original meeting.

We are grateful to all the participants for giving up time, and expending effort in preparing for and attending the meeting. In particular, we thank Professor Geoffrey Pearson for leading the discussions. Our thanks are also due to Mrs Lily Hughes, the Administrative Officer of the Society, for her excellent organization of the meeting.

London   M.L.
June 1991   G.E.
                                                                      D.C.D.

Contents

	List of contributors	ix
	List of invited discussants	x
1.	Problems and dependence: the history of two dimensions GRIFFITH EDWARDS	1
2.	Temperance cultures: concern about alcohol problems in Nordic and English-speaking cultures HARRY G. LEVINE	15
3.	Correlation and causality: notes on epistemological problems in substance abuse research OLE-JØRGEN SKOG	37
4.	Problems and dependence: chalk and cheese or bread and butter? D. COLIN DRUMMOND	61
5.	Substance-related problems in the context of international classificatory systems THOMAS F. BABOR	83
6.	Drinking problems: the individual in social context NORMAN KREITMAN	99
7.	The role of culture in the drug question GEOFFREY PEARSON	109
8.	Detecting individual factors in substance abuse problems LEE ROBINS	133
9.	Individual susceptibility to alcohol abuse and to ethanol toxicity TIMOTHY J. PETERS	151
10.	Problem definition: the case of the benzodiazepines MALCOLM LADER	161
11.	The problems perspective: implications for prevention policies REGINALD G. SMART	167

12. Treatment strategies within a problems framework
    D. COLIN DRUMMOND   179

13. The demands which the problem perspective sets for
    research
    MALCOLM LADER, GRIFFITH EDWARDS,
    and D. COLIN DRUMMOND   189

14. The meanings of problem: a debate around a problematic
    concept   199

    Index   211

Contributors to this book

T. F. BABOR, *The University of Connecticut Health Center, School of Medicine, Farmington, Connecticut 06032, USA.*

D. C. DRUMMOND, *Addiction Research Unit, National Addiction Centre, Institute of Psychiatry, University of London, UK.*

G. EDWARDS, *Addiction Research Unit, National Addiction Centre, Institute of Psychiatry, University of London, UK.*

N. KREITMAN, *MRC Unit for Epidemiological Studies in Psychiatry, Royal Edinburgh Hospital, Morningside Park, Edinburgh EH10 5HF, UK.*

M. LADER, *Section of Clinical Psychopharmacology, National Addiction Centre, Institute of Psychiatry, University of London, UK.*

H. G. LEVINE, *Department of Sociology, Queens College of City University of New York, Flushing, New York 11367, USA.*

G. PEARSON, *Goldsmiths' College, University of London, UK.*

T. J. PETERS, *Kings College of Medicine, Department of Clinical Biochemistry, Bessemer Road, London SE5 9PJ, UK.*

L. ROBINS, *Department of Psychiatry, Washington University School of Medicine, Washington University Medical Center, 4940 Audobon Avenue, St Louis, Missouri 63110, USA.*

O.-J. SKOG, *National Institute for Alcohol and Drug Research, Dannevigsvien 10, Oslo 4, Norway.*

R. G. SMART, *Prevention and Health Promotion Research and Development, Addiction Research Foundation, 33 Russell Street, Toronto, Ontario, Canada M5S 2S1.*

INVITED DISCUSSANTS AT THE 1990 CUMBERLAND LODGE MEETING

T. BEWLEY, *Royal College of Psychiatrists, 17 Belgrave Square, London SWIX 8PG, UK.*

H. GHODSE, *St George's Hospital Medical School, Section of Addictive Behaviour, Jenner Wing, Cranmer Terrace, London SW17 ORE, UK.*

B. HORE, *Alcoholism Treatment Unit, Withington Hospital, West Didsbury, Manchester M20 8LR, UK.*

T. KIDGER, *St Andrew's Hospital, Billing Road, Northampton NN1 5DG, UK.*

S. MACGREGOR, *Department of Politics and Sociology, Birkbeck College, Malet Street, London WC1E 7HX, UK.*

S. MADDEN, *The Countess of Chester Hospital, Priority and Community Services Unit, Liverpool Road, Chester CH2 1BQ, UK.*

L. MILBURN, *North West Regional Drug Training Unit, Kenyon Ward, Prestwich Hospital, Bury New Road, Manchester M25 7BL, UK.*

D. RAISTRICK, *Leeds Addiction Unit, 19 Springfield Mount, Leeds LS2 9NG, UK.*

J. RAVETZ, *The Council for Science and Society, 3/4 St Andrew's Hill, London EC4V 5BY, UK.*

D. TURNER, *Standing Conference on Drug Abuse, 1 Hatton Place, London EC1N 8ND, UK.*

J. WOODCOCK, *Institute for the Study of Drug Dependence, 1 Hatton Street, London EC1N 8ND, UK.*

Papers were presented at this meeting by D. Colin Drummond, Norman Kreitman, Harry G. Levine, Geoffrey Pearson, Timothy J. Peters, Duncan Raistrick, Lee Robins, and Ole-Jørgen Skog. They, Griffith Edwards, and Malcolm Lader also participated in the meeting.

1

Problems and dependence: the history of two dimensions

GRIFFITH EDWARDS

The first volume in the Society for the Study of Addiction's monograph series dealt with *The Nature of Drug Dependence* (Edwards and Lader 1990). With this second volume, the focus changes to *The Nature of Alcohol and Drug Related Problems*. Between them these two monographs explore a debate set within the framework proposed by a WHO report published in 1977 (Edwards *et al.* 1977). That report defined addiction as having two axes, dependence as one, and problems (or 'disabilities', to use the word employed in the original text) as the other.

This introductory chapter will examine the historical antecedents of the idea that 'dependence' and 'problems' are distinct and separable concepts. To the scholar who is familiar with the history of the ideas that affect this field, it will be evident that within the space available in a single book chapter, all that can be offered is a superficial mapping rather than any deep digging. Anyone who trespasses in this territory must confess their indebtedness to the general background of historical writings in this area, and especially to Virginia Berridge (Berridge and Edwards 1981; Berridge 1990), Harry Levine (Levine 1978, 1983), and David Musto (Musto 1973).

Most of the material taken to illustrate the arguments will relate to the history of alcohol rather than other drugs. That selectivity can be justified because for a long stretch of years the dominant drug problem encountered by the Western world was alcohol, and it was therefore around the attempt to understand the nature of drunkenness that the crucial developments in thinking took place. During the nineteenth century, the debate increasingly came to embrace the problems set by opium (Berridge and Edwards 1981), and in the mid-twentieth century, alcohol was for a time to be down-rated as an addictive drug because it did not fit the opiate paradigm (WHO 1952). At different points in history different substances have thus taken the lead role in shaping society's perceptions as to what really counts as addiction, or new substances have arrived to force some kind of partial revision — the benzodiazepines, and the issue they raise about the possibility of a 'normal dose dependence' provide just such a current example (see Chapter 10, p. 164).

'PROBLEMS' WERE RECOGNIZED LONG BEFORE 'DEPENDENCE'

For millenia, societies that used alcohol saw this substance as giving rise to problems. That assertion is true of ancient societies, of the Christian world from early times, of Buddhist cultures (de Silva 1983), and of Islamic societies, where one of the earliest religious ordinances involved the banning of intoxicants (Baasher 1983). The introduction of distilled spirits into Europe in the seventeenth century (Diethelm 1965), and the later widespread social disruption that stemmed from rapid urbanization and the socio-economic changes of the Industrial Revolution, exacerbated the anxieties of both State and Church about the drunkenness of the people (Shadwell 1902; Coffey 1966).

Until the middle of the eighteenth century, the only available way of thinking about this issue was as a set of particulate problems — blasphemy, swearing, stabbing, riot, neglect of family, collapse in the gutter — and the only explanation for the genesis of such egregious behaviour was in terms of the individual's sinfulness. If anyone had in those days talked about 'models' or 'path analysis', the prevalent model was very simple:

sinful choice → intoxication → disgraceful, dangerous, or ungodly behaviour.

THE BIRTH OF DEPENDENCE: DRUNKENNESS AS 'HABIT'

To suggest that a new model emerged as the result of any one individual contribution would be altogether too heroic. There was a ground swell of change (Porter 1985), and at some point during the eighteenth century a sharply different analysis of these issues began to be heard (Levine 1978). The astonishing break with the previous centuries (or millenia) of thinking, was the suggestion that the springs of habitual drunkenness lay not with the individual's sinfulness, but in his being in some sense disordered. Drunkenness, from being a sin, became a 'habit' or a 'disease'. That crucial transformation can only be understood when placed in the context of the eighteenth century Enlightenment, with its rationalism and respect for science, its rejection of religious authority, and the wider changes that were going on in medical thinking and practice.

Here is Boswell (Boswell 1791) giving a fascinating insight into the late eighteenth century thinking of a rational man:

September 16th 1773 ... he [Johnson] has great virtue in not drinking wine or any fermented liquor because as he acknowledged to us, he could not do it in moderation. Lady Macleod would hardly believe him and said 'I am sure, sir, you would not carry it too far.' Johnson, 'Nay, madam, it carried me. I took the opportunity of a long illness to leave if off; having broken off the habit, I have never returned to it.'

There is no suggestion in that passage that Johnson is repenting of a sin; he is breaking a habit, and that is a very different way of seeing things. By the time Boswell had opted for abstinence, the idea of drunkenness as habit had permeated quite widely into contemporary medicine. But if the roots of that concept lie in the ground swell of eighteenth century philosophical and medical thought, there can be no doubt that Benjamin Rush in America (Rush 1785), and Thomas Trotter in Britain (Trotter 1804), each made highly important individual contributions. Because they provided the first extended analyses of drunkenness in these new terms they fairly deserve the status of founding fathers. So far as the origins of the two dimensional dependence/problems model is concerned, they were, however, paying attention to both aspects, rather than focusing on the habit alone. Their keen awarenes of the significance of dependence, or, as Trotter put it, 'the evil genius of the habit itself', led both of them to theory-based proposals for individual treatment. The learnt habit had to be unlearnt, as exemplified in the following passage from Rush:

Our knowledge of the principle of association upon the minds and conducts of men, should lead us to destroy, by other impressions, the influence of all those circumstances, with which recollection and desire of spirits are combined ... Now by finding a new and interesting employment, or subject of conversation for drunkards, at the usual times in which they have been accustomed to drink ... their habits of intemperance can be completely destroyed.

As regards the problems dimension, Rush and Trotter were fully in the tradition of earlier medical writers (and preachers) in the emphasis they put on the consequence of drunkenness itself. Here, for instance, is a passage from Rush in which he lists what would much later be designated the social aspects of 'the problem dimension':

In pointing out the evils produced by ardent spirits, let us not pass by their effects upon the estates of the persons who are addicted to them. Are they inhabitants of cities? Behold! their houses stripped gradually of their furniture, and pawned, or sold by a constable to pay tavern debts ... Are they inhabitants of country places? Behold! their houses with shattered windows, — their barnes with leaky roofs, — their garden overrun with weeds, ... and their children filthy and half clad, without manners, principles, and morals.

Rush and Trotter were spared the invitation to put their thoughts into a path analysis, but retrospectively one can perhaps see their model thus. Alcohol, or, more particularly 'ardent spirits', was inherently addicting. Addiction was a disease of the will, a learned habit. That disease might lead to a wide array of problems or 'evils'. No categorical distinction was made between those drinkers who had or had not fallen victim to the habit, but the habit was seen as potentially insidious in its progression — as Rush put it, 'No man ever became suddenly a drunkard'. There could be problems without the fully developed habit.

Both Rush and Trotter used the words 'disease' as well as 'habit'. The linkage between the two concepts is made in Trotter's epigramatic statement 'The habit of drunkenness is a disease of the will'. The concept of 'habit' these writers were employing may have owed something to Hume and the early school of associationists, and it could be argued that their model of dependence derived from learning theory in a quite modern sense. However, it should at the same time be acknowledged that the concept of habit, and the meaning given to disease, must be seen as historically coloured. Although it is legitimate to trace important origins of later thinking to these writings, to take particular words out of historical context and assume identity with present-day usage would be careless in the extreme.

At this early but crucial phase in the evolution of ideas, however, it can certainly be seen that the word 'disease' was being trailed across the path. Both to interpret what was being said by Rush and Trotter at that time, and to head-off confusion when at a later period the 'disease concept' became prominent, it should be noted that concepts of 'disease' and 'habit' have at times become entangled, but are in reality conceptually distinct. Material we will shortly be considering will demonstrate that it is possible to view inebriety or alcoholism as a disease without conceiving of it as a habit. Furthermore, and as any present-day psychologist will argue, it is legitimate to view alcohol dependence as a habit without deeming it to be a disease. The history of what we are calling the dependence dimension is in large part a matter of trying to disentangle the evolution of ideas along an axis where at different points in history people have been talking about 'the habit of drunkenness', 'inebriety', 'dipsomania', 'the disease of alcoholism', or 'substance dependence'. 'Disease' ideas may at times have had within them an element of dependence ideas, but the two strands of thinking need to be distinguished.

It is paradoxical that twentieth century writers have often seen those two great eighteenth century contributors as founding fathers of 'the disease concept', when the texts suggest that their concept of disease was very different from that later employed by, say, Jellinek. This misreading becomes all the more extraordinary when one notes that these authors used 'habit' in a modern sense, and could therefore very properly be claimed as progenitors of a psychological view of dependence.

THE NINETEENTH CENTURY: INEBRIETY AS AN ORGANIZING IDEA

In the nineteenth century, Trotter and Rush were to be followed by a succession of medical writers (Bynum 1968), each of whom in turn made contributions to the elaboration of what we are calling here the 'dependence' dimension. Bruhl-Cramer in 1819 introduced the concept of *trunksucht* or drink-seeking, later to be given English translation as 'dipsomania'. Esquirol gave drunkenness its place within psychiatric classifications as a 'monomania' (Esquirol 1845). Magnus Huss (1849) coined the term 'alcoholismus'. In the latter part of the nineteenth century, a strong 'disease' school of alcoholism developed in both America (Crothers 1902) and Britain (Kerr 1888). These later writers promulgated 'inebriety' as an idea similar in many ways to the later generic concept of dependence: thus there could be inebriety relating to alcohol, opium, nicotine, coffee, chloroform, each being a variant on the generic theme. By now though, the disease that was being talked about was very different from a 'habit'. In tune with general trends in nineteenth century medicine it had become biologized and neurologized, with the added possibility of hereditary taint. There was likely to be something constitutionally wrong with the inebriate, a brain-cell vulnerability (hereditary or acquired), or an underlying and primary nervous disorder.

The disease concept of inebriety was a tool in campaigns for the opening of 'inebriate asylums' and similar institutions in both America and Britain. The doctors who were associated with this movement lobbied for the introduction of compulsory powers of detention for the treatment of sufferers from this alleged disease.

TEMPERANCE: ALCOHOL AS THE ROOT OF ALL EVIL

Intersecting with the disease concept of doctors, and their campaigns for institutional treatment and individual-directed solutions, was the nineteenth century Temperance movement (Gusfield 1963; Harrison 1971; Clark 1976). This movement placed strong emphasis on drink itself as the root cause of all manner of miseries, and emphasized the direct adverse consequences of alcohol as the forefront matters for concern. Temperance thus favoured a solution essentially at the public health level. It focused on the problem dimension, and at times Temperance advocates were frankly suspicious of a disease formulation, which might excuse the drunkard's behaviour and deflect attention from the need to attack alcohol as the source from which all consequent problems derived: the Temperance model did not require a disease as the intervening variable between 'drinking' and 'problems'. Here, for instance, is General Booth (1890), the founder of the Salvation Army, inveighing against alcohol in distinctly root and branch terms:

> Still the mighty torrent of Alcohol, fed by ten thousand manufactories, sweeps on, bearing with it, I have no hesitation in saying, the foulest, bloodiest tide that ever flowed from earth to eternity... We would to God that the temptation could be taken away from them, that every house licensed to send forth the black streams of bitter death were closed, and closed for ever.

Temperance writers not only spoke out on the need for individual abstinence and for society to be rid of alcohol, but to bolster their case produced a mass of statistics on the prevalence and cost of alcohol-related problems — one can see here the beginnings of a health economics approach. Baker (1896) wrote a book on the *Economics of the Drink Problem*, which subsequently went through numerous editions. In it he gave statistics on drinking and its impact on the family and on employment, and on its contribution to pauperism. He analysed 'The economic effect of drink-made crime upon the nation', and went on to quote Dr Hyslop as authority for the assertion that 'alcohol is either a direct or indirect factor in the causation of at least 50 per cent of the cases of insanity'.

The doctors, it could thus be argued, campaigned on a 'disease' platform, whereas the Temperance movement employed a 'problems' platform. To picture the doctors and the Temperance reformers as constituting sharply opposed parties would though be false. For instance, both Crothers and Kerr were personally committed to the Temperance cause: Crothers believed that all doctors had a duty to be total abstainers, and Kerr had set up a Temperance society while still a medical student at Glasgow. Furthermore, the Temperance workers were often able to combine their public health and problems stance with support for treatment campaigns, and the nature of the Temperance position changed over time.

THE TWENTIETH CENTURY AND THE DISEASE THEORY TRIUMPHANT

After the great debates of the nineteenth century, the early decades of the twentieth saw drunkenness become an issue of much less social importance than previously. In Britain the mean level of per capita alcohol consumption for the years 1925–29 was at exactly half the corresponding figure for 1890–94 (Royal College of Psychiatrists 1979): the combined influences of the Great War, Lloyd George, and economic slump, were making us a more temperate nation than any of the earlier Temperance workers could have envisaged. Meanwhile, in America the introduction of National Prohibition in 1919 appeared to make further investment in the study of alcoholism almost redundant, and with the coming of Repeal in 1933, alcohol remained a tainted topic from which sensible scientists stayed clear. The American Society for the Study of Addiction went out of existence (Blumberg 1978): the parallel British Society survived, but without much sense of purpose. The nineteenth century passions had been spent, and for several decades there were no great debates, no outstanding authorities, and certainly no further sustained attempt to delineate the nature of either the dependence or problems dimension.

The first signs of any considerable scientific reawakening of interest came with the steps that led within a few years to the establishment of the Yale Centre for Alcohol Studies. That story deserves fuller analysis, but it is probably correct to argue that its roots lay with a New York physician's interest in an aspect of the problem dimension — cirrhosis of the liver (Jolliffe 1936). Soon afterwards, both Strauss (see Strauss 1990) and Bacon (Bacon 1943, 1990) were breaking new ground in researching the relationship between drinking, homelessness, and crime — again, a focus on the problems perspective. But at much the same time Jellinek was developing an interest in 'alcohol addiction' (Bowman and Jellinek 1941), and with the publication of his report on 'Phases of alcohol addiction' (Jellinek 1952), Yale became the base for a re-launching of ideas that had been familiar to Kerr and Crothers (Lender 1979). Thus, over not much more than a decade, a gifted and energetic group of American scholars at one and the same time were forcing a reawakened concern for both the problems and dependence dimensions (Room 1990). The influence of Alcoholics Anonymous on Jellinek's thinking and his identification of 'loss of control' as the pathognomonic symptom of alcohol addiction should also be noted.

Jellinek was recruited to work on a literature review in 1939, moved to Yale in 1941, and then in 1950 moved to WHO headquarters in Geneva (Keller 1970), where he continued to be immensely influential. One may speculate that if it had been Strauss or Bacon who had relocated to Geneva with their sociological interests, history might have followed a different course. Jellinek showed an awareness of the public health aspects of drinking, but the questions around whether alcoholism was or was not a 'true addiction', and if so, the nature of that addiction, were issues that for a twenty year period undoubtedly held for him a greater and consuming interest. Through the agency of international seminars and a highly important series of WHO committees and their reports, Jellinek developed and refined his concept of alcoholism as addiction. Shortly after he left Geneva came the publication of the master work that was to secure his place in history, *The Disease Concept of Alcoholism* (Jellinek 1960).

So it came about that in the Anglo-Saxon world and by the 1960s, a new and pervasive consensus as to the nature of the drinking problem was established. The centrally important disorder was a physiological addiction to alcohol. Alcohol itself though was not the central issue: the drinker needed 'the X factor', some idiosyncratic predisposition (a neurosis, an allergy, or a hormonal imbalance), to render him or herself vulnerable to alcohol addiction.

Control of the liquor supply was therefore no part of the new enlightenment, and Prohibition was a mistaken experiment to be spoken of only with disparagement. Problems might occur without addiction (Jellinek's alpha and beta alcoholisms), but it was the addictive forms (delta, gamma, and perhaps epsilon) that were the true disease. The Jellinek model was:

an innately innocent agent → impact on vulnerable
and disease-prone individual → alcohol addiction and consequent problems.

And thus was the nineteenth century rediscovered. This was again the model of Kerr and Crothers in that it supported treatment campaigns (and AA), but it offered a wisdom that gave little place to prevention or the traditions of public health. The disease concept hijacked the dependence dimension: addiction was a biologized disease.

THE CONSENSUS CHALLENGED

We must return now to the WHO report on 'alcohol-related disabilities' (Edwards *et al.* 1977), which was mentioned briefly at the beginning of this chapter as explicitly defining the two dimensions of 'problems' and 'dependence'. That report radically challenged a consensus which at the time appeared to be immensely and confidently firm — alcoholism as categorical disease, and this disease the near exclusive focus for social activism and health programmes. Armed with the authority of WHO, there now however emerged an alternative view as to the true nature of the field of concern. The mapping of that field employed our two dimensions in the following way:

1. Great prominence was firstly given to the concept of 'alcohol-related disabilities'. Such a disability was 'deemed to exist when there is impairment in the physical, mental or social functioning of an individual, of such nature that it may be reasonably inferred that alcohol is part of the causal nexus determining the disability'. These disabilities (or problems) were recognized as public health concerns of pervasive importance in their own right, rather

than their being side-play to the great issue of 'the disease of alcoholism'. Thus, the report stated that:

... many individuals who experience disabilities related to alcohol consumption are not suffering from the dependence syndrome, and will not necessarily progress to that syndrome.

The multifarious nature of alcohol-related problems was underlined, the possibility of their varied clustering and severity noted, and attention was drawn to the fact that there might be much ebb and flow as individuals moved in and out of problem experience over time.

2. The alcohol dependence syndrome was described not as an all-or-none disease state, but as a condition which existed in degrees of severity:

The expositions of dependence in the prepared reviews were basically in terms of a learned phenomenon. If dependence is a learned behaviour, it may be expected to exist in various degrees of strength.

A formulation of 'learned phenomenon' existing in degrees thus conclusively embraced a dimensional as opposed to a categorical definition of the nature of what was being talked about. There was also an escape from definition of this dimension in disease terms: with emphasis given to the dimensionality of a *learned* phenomenon, the wheel had turned back full circle to 'habit'. On the use of the word 'disease', the report took the position that what does or does not count as disease is essentially a social issue:

The decision as to when a syndrome is to be designated a disease is in large measure socially determined, and must be congruent with wider cultural interests and habits: the syndrome formulation does not therefore undermine the position of those who have made the disease concept of alcoholism a central tenet of education and health-directed activism.

A question then arises as to the influences which conspired to bring about this shift in ways of thinking. The answers are probably several, but they can be grouped under two broad headings. Firstly, there was the impact of scientific developments which had taken place since the earlier consensus had been established. Under this heading can be identified, for instance, the work which was beginning to apply experimental methods to the study of drug-seeking behaviour within a learning paradigm (Stolerman and Goldberg 1986). Another relevant scientific input was the body of epidemiological investigation which was opening up an understanding of drinking practices and problems within the community, and which offered a different window than the hospital-based vision of alcoholism (Room 1977). Yet another type of research input related to the work which was convincingly demonstrating that population prevalence of drinking problems related to national per capita alcohol consumption (Bruun et al. 1975): it was difficult to square those findings with belief in an inevitable and pre-ordained disease. Suddenly any talk of 'factor X' or 'allergy' and the whole disease discourse which Jellinek had employed, appeared in scientific terms to be immensely irrelevant.

If science was one major catalyst for conceptual change, a second cluster of influences related to internationality. Thus, for instance, the French had never been keen on what they regarded as the mentalistic and redundant concept of 'alcoholism' (Pequignot 1990). For French scientists the focus had always been on the problems rather than addiction, and on the association between levels of drinking and level of harm. The report was also influenced by input from the Scandinavian tradition of alcohol studies which was rooted more in social science than in medicine (Bruun 1971).

HISTORY AND THE NEXT STEP FORWARD

As was stressed at the beginning of this chapter, what has been said here is intended only as a preliminary mapping of a difficult terrain. A heroic view of a report is likely to be as inaccurate and incomplete as the more familiar solipsism which exaggerates the role of the individual heroic actor. Furthermore, the 1977 report was very evidently only a further step in a long and continuing march, rather than a discovery of any New World. That report does though still provide a framework for some good questions. What, for instance, is a 'dimension' or an 'axis' really, and is this dressing up in the language of mathematics in part just a new disguise for ignorance? How do the two supposed dimensions relate to each other? Can problems be aggregated? Are problems really a commodity to be handled by science, or are they rooted essentially in socially determined and time-bound value judgements? These are just some of the questions which this book will seek to address.

Truly worthwhile historical inquiry directed at these issues cannot be conducted simply in terms of this or that contribution, or contributor, taken out of context. We have instead to address ourselves to why people thought as they did in 1790, 1890, in 1960, or in 1977, and try to understand the flow of background ideas which shaped the evolution of ideas in our particular area of concern. These questions relate to the general thought and temper of the time, the development of knowledge and theory within specific professions, and to communication between countries with historically and culturally embedded attitudes to alcohol and other drugs which have shown great diversity. Only with that kind of respect for depth and context can we expect history to throw light on why we think as we do today, and how to take the next step forward.

REFERENCES

Baasher, T. (1983). The use of drugs in the Islamic world. In Edwards, G., Arif, A., and Jaffe, J. (eds) *Drug use and misuse*, Chap. 2, pp. 21-32. Croom Helm, London.
Bacon, S. D. (1943). Sociology and the problems of alcohol: foundations for a sociologic study of drinking behaviour. *Quarterly Journal of Studies on Alcohol* **4**, 402-45.
Bacon, S. D. (1990). Interview with Selden Bacon. In Edwards, G. (ed.) *Addictions: personal influences and scientific movements*, Chap. 6, pp. 67-79. Transaction Publishers, New Brunswick.
Baker, J. J. (1896). *Economics of the drink problem*. Church of England Temperance Society, London.
Berridge, V. (1990). Special issue: The Society for the Study of Addiction 1884-1988. *British Journal of Addiction*, **85**, 983-1087.
Berridge, V. and Edwards, G. (1981). *Opium and the people*. Allen Lane, London.
Blumberg, L. (1978). The American Association for the Study and Cure of Inebriety. *Alcoholism: Clinical and Experimental Research*, **2**, 235-40.
Booth, General [William] (1890). *In darkest England and the way out*. International Headquarters of the Salvation Army, London.
Boswell, J. (1791). *Life of Johnson*. London.
Bowman, K. M. and Jellinek, E. M. (1941). Alcoholic mental disorders. *Quarterly Journal of Studies on Alcohol*, **2**, 312-90.
Bruhl-Cramer, C. von (1819). *Urber die Trunksucht und eine rationelle*. Heilmethode deserlben, Berlin.
Bruun, K. (1971). Finland: the non-medical approach. In Kiloh, L. G. and Bell, D. S. (eds) *Proceedings of the 29th International Congress on Alcoholism and Drug Dependence*, pp. 545-59. Butterworths, Sydney.
Bruun, K., Edwards, G., Lumio, M., Makela, K., Pan, L., Popham, R. E., Room, R., Schmidt, W., Skog, O.-J., Sulkunen, P., and Osterberg, E. (1975). *Alcohol control policies in public health perspective*. The Finnish Foundation for Alcohol Studies, Helsinki.
Bynum, W. F. (1968). Chronic alcoholism in the first half of the nineteenth century. *Bulletin of the History of Medicine*, **42**, 160-85.
Clark, N. H. (1976). *Deliver Us from Evil: An interpretation of American prohibition*. Norton, New York.
Coffey, T. G. (1966). Beer Street: Gin Lane: Some views of 18th century drinking. *Quarterly Journal of the Study of Alcohol*, **34**, 662-92.
Crothers, T. D. (1902). *Morphinism and narcomania from other Drugs. Their etiology, treatment and medico-legal relations*. W. B. Saunders, Philadelphia.
de Silva, P. (1983). The Buddhist attitude to alcoholism. In Edwards, G., Arif, A., and Jaffe, J. (eds) *Drug use and misuse*, Chap. 3, pp. 32-41, Croom Helm, London.
Diethelm, O. (1965). Chronic alcoholism of Northern Europe. *Akta Fracen Psychiatrie und Nurologie*, **2**, 29-30.

Edwards, G. and Lader, M. (eds) (1990) *The nature of drug dependence,* Society for the Study of Addiction Monograph No. 1. Oxford University Press, Oxford.

Edwards, G., Gross, M. M., Keller, M., Moser, J., and Room, R. (eds) (1977). *Alcohol-related Disabilities.* WHO, Geneva.

Esquirol, E. (1845). *Mental maladies treatise on insanity* (trans. from the French, with additions, by E. K. Hunt.) Lea and Blanchard, Philadelphia.

Gusfield, J. R. (1963). *Symbolic crusade: status policies and the American Temperance Movement.* University of Illinois Press, Urbana.

Harrison, B. (1971). *Drink and the Victorians.* Faber and Faber, London.

Huss, M. (1849). *Alcoholismus chronicus eller.* Chronisk Alkolssjukdom, Stockholm.

Jellinek, E. M. (1952). Phases of alcohol addiction. *Quarterly Journal of Studies on Alcohol,* **13**, 673–84.

Jellinek, E. M. (1960). *The disease concept of alcoholism.* Hillhouse, New Brunswick.

Jolliffe, N. (1936). The alcohol admissions to Bellevue Hospital. *Science,* **83**, 306–9.

Keller, E. M. (1970). Tribute to E. M. Jellinek. In Popham, R. E. (ed.) *Alcohol and alcoholism,* pp. xi–xvi. University of Toronto Press, Toronto.

Kerr. N. (1888). *Inebriety or narcomania. Its etiology, pathology, treatment and jurisprudence.* London: H. K. Lewis.

Lender, M. E. (1979). Jellinek's typology of alcoholism: some historical antecedents. *Quarterly Journal of Studies on Alcohol,* **46**, 361–75.

Levine, H. G. (1978). The discovery of addiction: changing conceptions of habitual drunkenness in America. *Journal of Studies on Alcohol,* **39**, 143–74.

Levine, H. G. (1983). Temperance and prohibition in America. In Edwards, G., Arif, A., and Jaffe, J. (eds) *Drug use and misuse,* Chap. 22, pp. 187–200. Croom Helm, London.

Musto, D. F. (1973). *The American Disease.* Yale University Press, New Haven.

Pequignot, G. (1990). Interview with George Pequignot. In Edwards, G. (ed.) *Addictions: personal influences and scientific movements,* Chap. 30, pp. 419–20. Transaction Publishers, New Brunswick.

Porter, R. (1985). The drinking man's disease: the pre-history of alcoholism in Great Britain. *British Journal of Addiction,* **80**, 385–96.

Room, R. (1977). Measurement and distribution of drinking patterns in general populations. In Edwards, G., Gross, M. M., Keller, M., Moser, J., and Room, R. (eds) *Alcohol related disabilities,* pp. 61–87. WHO, Geneva.

Room, R. (1990). Discussion starting on the fringe: studying alcohol in a wet generation. In Edwards, G. (ed.) *Addictions: personal influences and scientific movements,* Chap. 12, pp. 180–85. New Transaction Publishers, Brunswick.

Rush, B. N. (1785). *An enquiry into the effects of spiritous liquors on the human body.* Thomas and Andrews, Boston.

Royal College of Psychiatrists (1979). *Alcohol and alcoholism.* Tavistock, London.

Shadwell, A. (1902). *Drink, temperance and legislation.* Longmans Green, London.

Stolerman, I. P. and Goldberg, S. R. (eds) (1986). Introduction: brief history and scope of the behavioral approaches to dependence. In Goldberg, S. R. and

Stolerman, I. P. (eds) *Behavioral analysis of drug dependence*, Chap. 1. pp. 1–8. Academic Press, Orlando.

Strauss, R. (1990). Interview with Robert Strauss. In Edwards, G. (ed.) *Addictions: personal influences and scientific movements*, Chap. 7, pp. 81–103. Transaction Publishers, New Brunswick.

Trotter, T. (1804). *An essay, medical, philosophical and chemical, on drunkenness and its effects on the human body.* Longman, Hurst, Rees, and Orme, London.

World Health Organization (1952). *Expert Committee on Drugs Liable to Produce Addiction. Third Report*, Technical Report Series No. 57. WHO, Geneva.

2

Temperance cultures: concern about alcohol problems in Nordic and English-speaking cultures

HARRY G. LEVINE

INTRODUCTION

This book deals with 'problems.' Historians and sociologists studying the history of ideas often take as their starting point the observation that objective conditions by themselves are not sufficient to produce a definition of something as a social or public problem (Mills 1959). Even in modern societies, many undesirable, unhealthy or dangerous behaviours and conditions exist for long periods of time without becoming the focus of social movements or government action. In the US, air and water pollution, automobile design, and hand-gun murders, to choose only three examples, long generated no public interest or outcry. One cannot explain from objective conditions, from the existence of real-life problems and suffering, why in America men and women who had an alcoholic parent have organized themselves into a sizeable self-help movement (called 'Adult Children of Alcoholics'), or why, say, those who grew up with a parent who battered them have not. One cannot explain from objective conditions why there are no groups called 'Adult Children of the Mentally Ill' or 'Adult Children of the Poor.'

There is no doubt that alcohol is a powerful consciousness-altering substance that is easily and frequently misused; yet only some societies in the nineteenth or early twentieth centuries organized large ongoing temperance movements concerned with the dangers and evils of alcoholic drink — with alcohol problems. In fact, only some of the societies that experienced considerable amounts of drunkenness developed major movements focused on alcohol problems. Even today only some societies retain a strong concern with alcohol problems and alcohol misuse (or abuse).

This chapter results from an effort to determine those societies (such as the US, UK, and Finland) that developed large, ongoing temperance movements in the nineteenth and early twentieth centuries, and those (such as Italy, France, and Belgium) that did not. Unfortunately, there are no cross-cultural studies of temperance movements to turn to; the field of comparative temperance studies does not yet exist. However, the recent growth of the field of social history, and of scholarly interest in temperance movements, and the rich supply of primary temperance documents, make it possible to identify (with some certainty) those places that did have major movements concerned with alcohol problems.

This chapter first reports some results of a search for a kind of 'historical taxonomy' of temperance. *The term temperance cultures is used here to refer to those societies which, in the nineteenth and early twentieth centuries, had large, enduring temperance movements.* There were nine of these temperance cultures: the English-speaking cultures of the US, Canada, the UK, Australia, and New Zealand; and the northern Scandinavian or Nordic societies of Finland, Sweden, Norway, and Iceland. Some of the temperance cultures still have active versions of the old temperance organizations. In temperance cultures, the movement's concerns about the dangers of alcoholic drink — about alcohol problems — extended far beyond formal membership and achieved widespread acceptance and legitimacy in the larger society.

Having identified these Nordic and English-speaking societies as the temperance cultures, the obvious question is: can we determine anything distinctive about them all, as compared with non-temperance cultures, that might help explain why they developed major temperance movements? This is obviously a huge topic.

As Eriksen (1990) points out, much research in recent years, especially in Europe, has tended to focus on political and economic factors contributing to temperance. To some extent, temperance was associated almost everywhere with economic change, industrialization, and social protest. In temperance cultures, significant numbers of large employers and wealthy merchants, as well as much of the middle class, tended to support temperance. In some places there was also considerable working class participation, especially from the 'labour aristocracy.' Temperance was also involved in national, regional, and ethnic conflicts. There may have been something common about the political economy of societies as diverse as the UK, Finland, Australia, the US, and Sweden that distinguishes them from non-temperance cultures. But there may not have been. It is just not possible at this early stage of historical and sociological scholarship to determine what, if anything, is unique about the political economy of temperance cultures. In this chapter, therefore, we look at other issues.

We will discuss two factors that do strongly correlate with temperance activity. First, people in temperance cultures drank a considerable portion of their alcohol in distilled liquor (mainly vodka, gin, rum, or whiskey). Second, all the temperance cultures were predominantly Protestant societies.

The first section develops the taxonomy of temperance activity and discusses the differences between temperance and non-temperance cultures. That basic historical classification is probably the most important finding reported in this chapter. The second section discusses whether drunkenness and disruption can account for temperance activity. It then explores the relationship of temperance movements to Protestantism as a culture, and focuses on the importance of self-restraint as an issue for Protestantism and for temperance movements.

The final section extends the discussion about temperance cultures into the present. It offers a rough test of the (perhaps intuitive) hypothesis that the societies which had large. temperance movements in the past also retain the strongest concern with alcohol misuse (abuse) and alcohol problems. It does this by comparing the membership figures for Alcoholics Anonymous in a number of Western countries. It finds, perhaps not surprisingly, that the strongest centres of Alcoholics Anonymous membership in Western societies are among the temperance cultures.

This chapter outlines some in progress findings and conclusions, from my own research and from that of other historians and social scientists, in the hope of contributing to a growing international conversation about the history and sociology of movements and ideas about alcohol problems. It is not the final word.

TEMPERANCE CULTURES

In Western societies, only Nordic and English-speaking cultures developed large, ongoing, extremely popular temperance movements in the nineteenth century and the first third or so of the twentieth century. Table 2.1 lists 24 Western cultures; 15 of them were *not* temperance cultures. A more complete list would include Yugoslavia, and the Soviet Union's Western republics (such as the Ukraine) identified individually. In other words, there are even more non-temperance cultures than the table indicates. (See the entries for different countries in Cherrington's remarkable five volume *Encyclopedia of the Liquor Problem* (1924–30);[1] For individual societies also see: Gusfield 1988; Blocker 1989; Paulson 1973; Levine 1984; Harrison 1971; Malcolm 1986; Bengtsson 1938; Eriksen 1990; Room 1988, 1989,

---

[1] Cherrington was a life-long leader in the temperance and prohibitionist movements. He tended to report any temperance activity he could find, and his *Encyclopedia of The Alcohol Problem* should be read as the work of an inveterate movement booster. Nonetheless, Cherrington's *Encyclopedia* is an invaluable work and the best single source on the character of temperance in difference countries. Also see the discussions of Cherrington in Kerr (1985) and in Lender (1984).

TABLE 2.1 Apparent consumption of alcohol for the population age 15 years and over in 24 Western countries, in litres per capita for 1974 and 1984

	Litres per capita absolute alcohol from all drinks 1974	1984	Per cent spirits of all alcohol 1974	1984	Per cent wine of all alcohol 1974	Per cent beer of all alcohol 1974	AA groups per million persons 1986
1. Iceland*	4.9	5.5	72.7	54.5	11.0	16.1	high†
2. Norway*	5.5	5.2	43.0	32.6	10.2	46.7	16.8
3. Sweden*	6.9	6.4	47.4	41.6	16.2	36.2	11.1
4. Finland*	7.6	8.2	51.7	44.9	10.9	37.3	103.4
5. Poland	8.0	8.2	67.2	67.0	15.7	16.9	0.4
6. Ireland	8.3	9.7	30.0	22.6	5.2	64.6	136.0
7. United Kingdom*	10.1	9.2	19.8	21.7	14.7	65.3	39.5
8. United States*	10.4	10.2	41.1	35.2	12.0	46.8	123.5
9. Netherlands	10.6	11.0	34.0	27.2	22.2	43.0	124
10. Canada*	10.7	10.2	35.6	33.3	11.2	53.1	163.9
11. Denmark	10.9	12.9	20.2	14.7	19.1	60.5	0.6
12. Soviet Union	11.8‡	11.5	62.3	67.8	28.1	8.9	0
13. Czechoslovakia	11.2	13.5	30.8	31.8	19.0	49.2	0

14. Hungary	12.3	14.6	30.9	43.1	45.0	21.9	0
15. New Zealand*†	12.6	11.0	14.5	22.7	14.9	70.4	75.9
16. Spain	12.8	15.0	25.2	26.0	73.0	1.7	4.6
17. Australia*†	13.2	12.5	13.3	12.8	18.0	68.6	59.6
18. Italy	13.5	15.1	9.2	10.5	84.7	5.7	2.4
19. Switzerland	13.9	13.9	20.4	18.7	44.0	35.4	23.1
20. Austria	14.0	14.3	22.5	13.2	33.5	43.9	0
21. Belgium	14.3	13.3	16.0	18.0	19.4	64.5	54.8
22. West Germany	14.8	14.3	23.2	19.5	19.9	56.8	30.1
23. France	22.4	18.2	19.6	11.7	66.3	13.9	4.6
24. Portugal	23.4	17.8	3.2	6.1	88.7	7.8	0.6

* Indicates a temperance culture.

Sources:

For 1974: Adapted and computed from Mark Keller and Carol Gurioli (1976). Statistics on consumption of alcohol and on alcoholism. *Journal of Studies on Alcohol* p. 10.

For 1984: Adapted and computed from Marc Eliany (1989). *Alcohol in Canada*. Minister of Supply and Services, Canada.

For AA figures: Klaus Mäkelä. Social and cultural preconditions of AA and factors associated with the strength of AA, Presented at Kettil Bruun Society for Social and Epidemiological Research on Alcohol, Budapest, 3–8 June, 1990.

† Mäkelä did not compute a AA per million persons figure for Iceland. However it is by far the country with the highest per capita AA membership in the world.

‡ Includes estimated home-made drinks.

1990; de Lint 1981; Sulkunen 1986; Vogt 1981; Alasuutari 1990; Roberts 1984; Prestwich 1988; Smith and Christian 1984).

Temperance cultures, it is important to note, are not the heaviest drinkers. In fact, temperance nations today consume significantly *less* pure alcohol per capita than most non-temperance societies (See Table 2.1).

However, temperance cultures do have a distinctive drinking pattern. People in temperance cultures drink a substantial portion of their alcohol in distilled liquors, or did so during the formative periods of their temperance crusade. In recent decades, spirits consumption has declined among some of these countries. Nonetheless, most temperance cultures still consume a significant portion of their alcohol in hard liquors. In 1974, for example, the US consumed 41 per cent of its alcohol in distilled liquor, Canada 35 per cent, Finland, Norway and Sweden all averaged between 43 and 51 per cent. Iceland, which leads the world in per capita membership in Alcoholics Anonymous, consumed a remarkable 72 per cent of its alcohol in distilled drinks. See Table 2.1 for complete figures. The UK today has a much lower level of spirits consumption, about 20 per cent; Australia and New Zealand are even lower. However, in the nineteenth century when the temperance campaign was stronger in Britain, Australia, and New Zealand, spirits consumption was much higher (Room 1988; Harrison 1971; Cherrington 1924–30).

The other common characteristic of temperance cultures is that they were all predominately Protestant societies. Temperance cultures are places where Protestantism historically shaped psychology and culture, and where the dominant or state religion has been a version of Protestantism.

Non-temperance cultures, places that did not develop large temperance movements, typically lacked either a Protestant tradition, or a pattern of distilled liquor drinking, or both. Of the two factors, Protestantism appears to have been more important for the development of temperance movements. Small versions of classic temperance movements did develop among Protestants in Denmark, Holland, Switzerland, and Germany. On the other hand, even small-scale enduring temperance organizations did not develop to nearly the same extent in non-Protestant societies — even those with high levels of hard-liquor consumption such as Russia and Poland (Eriksen 1990; de Lint 1981; Roberts 1984; Smith and Christian 1984; Cherrington 1924–30).

Occasionally the non-Protestant, hard-liquor drinking societies have developed anti-drunkenness campaigns usually led by an economic, political, or religious elite. These anti-drunkenness crusades have tended to be sporadic and isolated affairs; they have aimed at mobilizing the population for economic, political, or religious reform, but have soon exhausted themselves and generally left behind no developed organization or ongoing movement. Recently, for example, the Soviet Union under Gorbachev's direction launched the most dramatic and large scale elite-sponsored anti-drunkenness campaign ever attempted in a non-Protestant country (Partanen 1987). That crusade, which was primarily an effort to instill a new, more disciplined work ethic, quickly collapsed like earlier ones in the face of an indifferent-to-hostile public reaction.

The most famous nineteenth century temperance crusade in a non-Protestant culture was that of Father Mathew in Ireland in the 1840s. As Malcolm (1986) makes clear in her recent excellent study of Irish temperance, *Ireland Free, Ireland Sober*, Father Mathew's crusade was the sole important moment of Catholic temperance in nineteenth century Ireland, and it left behind little in the way of ongoing organization or movement. Malcolm reports that Irish temperance began, with impetus from American temperance reformers, as the work of evangelical Protestants in Ulster and then of Quakers in Dublin. She traces the meteoric rise and fall of Father Mathew's campaign in the 1840s. Irish Protestants, on the other hand, did organize large successful temperance organizations. Yet, despite all their efforts, and despite Father Mathew's fame, in the nineteenth century Irish Catholics could not by and large be persuaded to take up the temperance cause. It was only after 70 years of sustained Protestant temperance proselytizing, and the work of another skilled Irish Catholic temperance organizer, that the Pioneer Total Abstinence Association was established. It seems reasonable to conclude that, were it not for British and Irish Protestant temperance groups, temperance would have had even less impact on Ireland. (Also see the brief discussion of Irish temperance in Cherrington 1926.)

At the far non-temperance end of the spectrum are the predominately Catholic wine-drinking societies. There was little if any temperance activity in wine-drinking cultures such as Italy, France, Spain, Portugal, Greece, Romania, and Austria. People in wine-drinking cultures do not commonly hold negative views of alcohol even though they consume two to four times more pure alcohol per capita than do the spirit drinking Nordic countries (roughly 12–18 litres of pure alcohol per capita for wine cultures vs 5–8 litres in the Nordic Countries (see Table 2.1). Men and women in wine cultures still regard alcohol chiefly as a food, and rarely focus on it as a significant cause of economic or social problems. In wine cultures, alcoholic drink does not have strong negative symbolic meanings — indeed, wine is overwhelmingly imbued with positive symbolic meaning. (Lolli *et al.* 1958; Sadoun *et al.* 1965).

In the nineteenth and early twentieth centuries there was certainly temperance activity outside of the English-speaking and Nordic countries. As noted above, Denmark, the Netherlands, Switzerland, and Germany all had active temperance movements and organizations. There were some people in those countries who regarded alcohol in much the same way as many people did in the Nordic and English-speaking countries. Alcohol policy was debated in legislatures and by political parties, especially by Social Democrats. The key difference between between these non-temperance countries and the temperance cultures is that in the latter societies the anti-alcohol movements had much greater legitimacy, influence, and popular acceptance — they were more mainstream. In the Nordic and English-speaking cultures a much larger percentage of the population came to accept the basic ideas or message of temperance (and more of the upper-classes or elites did as well). This quantitative difference constituted, over time, a real qualitative difference between temperance and non-temperance cultures.

All temperance movements had high and low periods. In the Nordic and English-speaking cultures, organizations held on during the low times; in the non-temperance cultures they tended to disappear. Thus in the 1920s, when Cherrington wrote his *Encyclopedia of the Alcohol Problem*, he celebrated the triumph or potential triumph of prohibitionism in a number of Nordic and English-speaking countries. However, when writing about Germany he was forced to wonder where the once active organizations and movements had gone.

LIQUOR, PROTESTANTISM, SELF-CONTROL, AND TEMPERANCE

Spirit drinking and disruption

Distilled liquor makes drunkenness easier and more likely. It seems relatively clear, therefore, why hard-liquor drinking, especially when coupled with a pattern of drinking to drunkenness, is correlated with temperance activity. In all the original temperance cultures, gin, vodka, rum, or whisky produced the drunkenness that anti-drink campaigns took as their original enemy (Rorabaugh 1979; Harrison 1971; Eriksen 1990; Sulkunen 1986; Room 1988; Alasuutari 1990). The public drunkard — staggering, vomiting, and dishevelled — offered the visible evidence of the evils of alcohol that temperance crusades drew upon in their ideology and imagery (Lender and Karnchanapee 1977; Levine 1978, 1980, 1983).

Several readers of an earlier version of this chapter suggested that the disruptions that spirit-drinking caused might have been sufficient to explain the presence of temperance movements. For example, in a perceptive and helpful set of comments, Klaus Mäkelä accepted this chapter's general argument about the taxonomy of temperance cultures in the Nordic and English-speaking cultures. Mäkelä also proposed that temperance activity was caused by a kind of drinking which actually did pose 'an objective threat to social order'. Let us term this 'the disruption hypothesis'.

Despite its intuitive appeal (especially from within a temperance culture), for both empirical and conceptual reasons, the disruption hypothesis cannot by itself explain the rise of temperance movements. First of all, a drinking pattern that included getting very drunk on hard liquor (vodka) did not produce large scale temperance movements in Russia and Poland. The Russians and Poles were certainly not more moderate drinkers, for example, than Swedes or Norwegians. And there is no evidence that the social disruption caused by spirit drinking was greater among Swedes and Norwegians than among Russians and Poles. The absence of the Russians and Poles from the ranks of the cultures that developed large, enduring temperance movements means that the personal and social disruptions caused by drunkenness from hard liquor did not, by themselves, produce the movements.

Second, the disruption hypothesis does not address the enormous shift in morals and perception necessary for the rise of anti-drink consciousness. Massive public drunkenness had been common for several thousand years without generating much moral opprobrium. In the US, heavy spirit-drinking leading to drunkenness existed for a hundred years before a temperance movement arose. As a number of writers have observed (Tyrell 1979; Levine 1978, 1983; Alasuutari 1990), the temperance movement was part of a much larger cultural transformation in values. These changes included, for example: the condemnation of torture and the rise of 'humane' punishment and prisons (Foucault 1977); the rejection of the idea that insanity reduced people to animals, and the embrace of the idea of mental disease (Foucault 1965); new attitudes about the special character of children and childhood (Aries 1962); a new attention to and loquaciousness about sexuality (Foucault 1978) — and, in addition to many other shifts, the increased legitimacy of democratic values.

Even if we accept as scientifically true everything that nineteenth century temperance advocates said about the dangers of alcohol and the disruptions it caused, we still need to explain what enabled so many people in the nineteenth century to finally *see* the 'truth' about alcohol. In short, a recognition that spirits drinking easily led to drunkenness does not eliminate the need for a social or cultural explanation of the new perceptions about drink, and of the new moral standards about drunkenness.

In his rich and insightful study, *Drink, Temperance and the Working class in Nineteenth-Century Germany* (1984), James Roberts points out that even when Germans drank spirits they tended to consume small amounts all day long; they drank it with food, and as a high calorie but less bulky substitute for potatoes and bread. Despite such a relatively undisruptive drinking style, Germany developed a moderate sized, influential temperance movement. This Protestant dominated temperance movement in Germany was larger and more mainstream than the temperance movement in Russia.

And the German temperance reformers worried about drunken disorder even though, compared to Russians, they did not see that much of it (Smith and Christian 1984; Cherrington 1924–30).

Similarly, in Protestant Switzerland, despite a tradition of beer and wine drinking without much drunkenness, the temperance movement endures to this day. For example, in 1986 at a public health conference on alcohol and drugs in Vienna, the author met two Swiss ladies who were active members of a Women's Christian Temperance Union chapter. Indeed, the connection between Protestantism and temperance is so strong that it is unusual to find a Protestant culture without at least some small classic temperance activity.

Protestantism, temperance and self-control

There is no doubt that a number of different factors contributed to the making of large-scale temperance movements. The beginning of this chapter observed that a type of industrial or capitalist political-economy, a stage of economic development, or perhaps even a kind of family pattern, may have contributed to the rise of large temperance movements. However, without excluding other factors, the author would like to briefly suggest the outlines of an argument about why the correlation between temperance activity and Protestantism should not be viewed as a coincidence.

In the last forty years, religion has not served as a major focus for social scientific inquiry, but in the early twentieth century the situation was rather different. At that time a number of social scientists — notably Emile Durkheim, Max Weber, Bronislaw Malinowski, and Sigmund Freud — viewed religion as a social and cultural variable which was necessary for understanding fundamental areas of individual and social life. Weber and Durkheim are especially relevant for our discussion because they focused on Protestantism and understood it in a broadly cultural or strongly anthropological sense. Clifford Geertz has captured this perspective well in his notion (and discussion) of 'Religion as a cultural system' (Geertz 1973). Viewed in this way, Protestantism is not merely a set of theological beliefs, but rather a social psychology, a system of sacred and secular symbols, a pattern of social and institutional relationships and expectations — it is norms, values, institutions and, to some extent personality.

In his classic study *Suicide* (1951), Durkheim maintained that the different rates of suicide among Protestants, Catholics, and Jews — with the Protestants having the highest and Jews the lowest — was not a coincidence but followed from real social and cultural differences among the groups. In *The Protestant Ethic and the Spirit of Capitalism* (1958), Weber made much the same sociological point about the strong relationship between ascetic Protestantism and early capitalist activity.

Both sociologists focused on the question of self-regulation and control.

According to Durkheim, the 'religious individualism' of Protestantism produced a culture in which norms emphasized self-sufficiency and self-control, and in which people actually were less regulated by other people. According to Weber, the 'worldly asceticism' of Protestantism produced a psychology which stressed the importance of self-regulation and self-restraint.

Weber and Durkheim saw this emphasis on self-control, over more external or collective forms of control, as characteristic of modernizing societies in general and of Protestant ones in particular. Weber stressed the affinity between Protestantism and modern capitalism; both Protestantism and early capitalist business demanded that the individual subject himself 'to the supremacy of a purposeful will, to bring his actions under constant self-control'. Durkheim focused on the social pathologies that Protestant and modern cultures produced: they both freed people from external restraints thereby producing 'egoism', and they weakened the moral influence of other people thus producing 'anomie'.

In keeping with Weber and Durkheim's analysis, this chapter suggests that temperance movements successfully appealed to and mobilized people in modern, Protestant cultures because the movements had found an ideological and organizational way of addressing this central concern with self-discipline and regulation. In the Nordic and English-speaking cultures — indeed, in any place where temperance movements developed — alcohol was defined as dangerous, as a problem, in terms of its perceived ability to destroy individual self-control. Alcohol became a focus for concerns and anxieties (both real and imaginary) about individual self-control.

The name of the movement provides a major clue to understanding its appeal. Historians and journalists have sometimes been confused by the name of the nineteenth century alcohol movement because they believed that 'temperance' was the wrong name for what (in America) was largely a crusade for total abstinence. But temperance movement advocates always insisted that it was the perfect name because *temperance means self-control*. From the early nineteenth century on, they argued that alcohol was dangerous and destructive precisely because it destroyed drinkers' ability to regulate their own behaviour. The whole temperance crusade was built upon a now 200-year-old reinterpretation of the effect of alcohol that centred on its capacity to weaken and destroy self-control and self-discipline (Levine 1978, 1983).

According to temperance speakers and writers, alcohol weakened the 'higher' and moral portions of the brain and personality and, they asserted, it took very little alcohol to do this. Although wine drinkers in Italy and other Catholic countries did not tend to view alcohol as a dangerous stimulant to aggressive or violent behaviour, Protestant spirit drinkers, and even some Protestants in beer cultures, did view alcohol in this way.

Temperance supporters in the nineteenth century also maintained that alcohol was an inherently addicting drug (the way people often think of heroin today), and that it eventually enslaved most drinkers. Even though Catholic wine drinkers (for example, in Italy and France) consumed more alcohol more often than Protestant spirit drinkers (in Norway and Sweden) — and as a result still have substantially higher rates of liver cirrhosis — it was the Protestants who focused on the 'addicting' character of alcohol and talked about long term use producing a 'disease of the will'. The wine drinkers have higher mortality from heavy use, but the Protestant spirit drinkers talk much more about addiction.

In short, just as Durkheim and Weber found Protestantism empirically correlated with what they were studying (suicide and capitalist activity), so too was it correlated with the presence of large, ongoing temperance movements. And just as Durkheim and Weber found that the association was not coincidental, so too was that the case with temperance movements. And finally, just as Durkheim and Weber insisted that the high levels of Protestant suicide and capitalist activity needed to be understood partly as a result of Protestantism's institutional, conceptual, and psychological emphasis on the issues of individual autonomy and self-control, so too was that the case for the temperance movement.

Temperance movements have, since the nineteenth century, focused on self-control. People in Protestant cultures found alcohol to be such a compelling social issue, in large part because its effects were interpreted so as to focus individual and collective attention onto questions of self-control and self-discipline. Self-control is the key social-psychological problem addressed both by classic temperance movements and by contemporary alcohol problem movements.

The concern with self-control is of course not limited to temperance movements or Protestant cultures. As Weber, Freud, Elias and many other scholars have observed, *self-control is a central psychological problem with which all modern peoples and societies must struggle.* The weakening of traditional forms of regulation and control (and the increase in freedom of all sorts) require that all modern peoples must continually deal with the problem of self-regulation. *However, some cultures, notably Protestantism, further emphasized individual moral responsibility for personal behaviour.* All modern cultures to some extent now see alcohol as raising problems of self-restraint. However, some Western cultures have made much more of it, emphasized it more, and in the nineteenth and early twentieth centuries, supported large ongoing movements and ideologies concerned with alcohol as a special and important problem of self-regulation. These are all Protestant cultures which traditionally drank a substantial portion of their alcohol in distilled liquor. These are the temperance cultures.

One last point: most Protestant spirit-drinking societies developed large temperance movements. But not all of them did, as Sidel Eriksen (1990) has recently pointed out in a superb piece of historical sociology. In the nineteenth and early twentieth centuries, Danes consumed great quantities of distilled liquor. They had plenty of drunkenness, disruption, Protestantism, and industrial dislocation. But, compared to Sweden, they had relatively little temperance movement activity. Why? Eriksen's answer is that Sweden and Denmark had different kinds of Protestantism. Or, more precisely, Sweden developed a Christian revival movement strongly influenced by 'Anglo-American revivalism' whereas 'the Danish revivalist movement of the same period' was pietistic and Lutheran.

Eriksen traces the roots of Swedish temperance directly to Anglo–American bible societies and to Methodist and Baptist missionary organizations. These are also precisely the groups that provided the backbone of temperance support in the US, and along with other dissenting groups like Presbyterians and Quakers, in Canada, Australia, and the UK. Denmark's Lutheran pietists, on the other hand, generally opposed the temperance campaign. During the nineteenth century, Methodist and Baptist missionaries made little headway in Denmark, and therefore so did temperance. Only after 1901, writes Eriksen, 'did the Methodist inspired currents in Inner Mission gain ground, leading to the creation of the Christian temperance associations, the Blue Cross, with several local affiliates around the countryside. Yet the organization was hardly accepted by all Inner Mission circles, and it never succeeded in influencing public opinion'.

It is impossible to do justice here to the detail of Eriksen's analysis which closely follows the development of Swedish and Danish religious revivals and temperance movements. It also distinguishes, in good Weberian fashion, between the world view of Lutheran Pietism and that of Anglo-American revivalists highlighting the characteristics which made the latter so keen on temperance, and the former opposed to it. Eriksen's paper became available just as this chapter was going to press. Any further exploration of the social sources of concern with alcohol problems in the nineteenth and early twentieth centuries, and of the character of temperance cultures, must now begin with Eriksen's argument about the very strong relationship between temperance sentiment and what she terms 'Anglo–American Protestantism.' In conclusion, Eriksen's research suggests that we might conceptualize religious proclivity or openness for temperance along a continuum: Roman Catholics and the various forms of Orthodox and Eastern religious cultures would be at one end; pietistic Lutheran cultures would occupy a more middle position; and the dissenting churches of Anglo–American Protestantism would tend to make the strongest temperance supporters.

THE SPREAD AND LIMITS OF TEMPERANCE CULTURE

Since the early 1800s, the US has been at the forefront of temperance crusades. In the nineteenth century, American temperance ideas spread to the British and Nordic countries where groups like the Women's Christian Temperance Union and the Good Templars developed active chapters. The prohibition movement was strongest in America, which was the only Western country, other than Finland, to institute complete national alcohol prohibition.

The main American export of the last fifty years has been Alcoholics Anonymous and the disease concept of alcoholism. In the 1930s, two middle class men from New England created Alcoholics Anonymous by combining elements from evangelical Christianity, with themes from twentieth century psychology and psychoanalysis, and with some of the basic elements of nineteenth century temperance thought and organizations (Kurtz 1979). In so doing they created what is surely the most important American alcohol organization of the twentieth century, and a distinctive, new movement concerned with alcohol problems (Denzin 1987).

In part, American ideas have been so influential because its alcohol movements and efforts have been comparatively well organized and well funded. In addition, Alcoholics Anonymous (like nineteenth century temperance) has a strong missionary element, which it carries over from its evangelical Christian roots. AA teaches recovering alcoholics that their sobriety depends upon bringing the message of AA to others through 'Twelfth Step work.' Finally, in the period since the Second World War, the enormous economic, political, and military powers of the US have also increased the international influence of American culture on many issues including views of alcohol and drugs.

In the last ten or fifteen years the US has witnessed a resurgence of public concern with drinking, and a growing variety of popular new alcohol organizations and movements, that many observers have rightly termed new temperance or neo-temperance. Chief among the developments has been the spread of the philosophy of AA and the appearance and rapid growth of related groups notably Adult Children of Alcoholics (ACoA). Perhaps the other most important alcohol problem organization has been MADD (Mothers Against Drunk Drivers) and its spin-off SADD (Students Against Drunk Driving). Though not as obviously linked to classic temperance concerns, MADD has in fact organized around a theme central to earlier temperance crusades: the defence of women, children, and the family from dangerous, drunken men (Reinarman 1988; Levine 1980; Epstein 1981). Francis Willard, the long time head of the Women's Christian

Temperance Union, would certainly have approved of Adult Children of Alcoholics and of MADD and SADD.

One motivation for developing the taxonomy of temperance and non-temperance cultures presented in this paper was to use it in making sense of current movements and activities concerned with alcohol problems. In America, at least, current alcohol movements draw upon themes and images that have been central to earlier temperance organizations. My informal hypothesis, from over fifteen years observing the alcohol field, has been that in recent years, popular and scientific concern with alcohol problems has been strongest among the English-speaking and Nordic countries. For example, it is those nations that send most of the scientists and researchers to international collaborative studies on alcohol problems and policy. However, it is difficult to statistically test the idea that societies which have had large temperance movements in the past have retained the strongest concern with alcohol problems and misuse. Some of the more recent American new temperance groups such as MADD or ACoA have not spread very much outside of the US.

Alcoholics Anonymous, on the other hand, has established itself in other countries. Indeed, AA today is described in the American mass media as a world-wide movement with meetings and members in many countries. AA membership reports, a limited amount of other formal research, and a substantial amount of anecdotal data suggest that AA and the larger alcoholism movement have grown steadily in the US and in other temperance cultures (Leach and Norris 1977; Mäkelä 1990). AA membership data, collected and computed by Mäkelä, allows us to compare AA membership in 24 of the Western cultures we have been discussing in this paper.

There is good reason to view with scepticism claims about the universal appeal of American movements and ideologies. Leach and Norris (1977) found that the number of AA groups per million people in Canada and Australia about equalled (or at times even exceeded) that of the US from 1945 to 1970. In the UK, however, the number of AA groups per capita remained much lower than in the other English-speaking regions. AA membership has also grown substantially in the Nordic countries, especially Finland. Yet even in Finland, Alcoholics Anonymous is still only one of several available forms of treatment, and it accounts for only a minority of such efforts. Most Finns with drinking problems still turn to the national health-care system, to the network of A-Clinics which use a variety of psychotherapeutic approaches, and to the indigenous Finnish self-help movement called A-Guilds (Alasuutari 1990). This is the opposite of the situation in the US where the philosophy of AA — of the twelve-step movement — dominates in-patient and out-patient treatment, therapeutic communities, and nearly all drug self-help groups. Further, alcoholism treatment in most European countries — both temperance and non-temperance

30 *The Nature of Alcohol and Drug Related Problems*

— allows for moderate drinking — a notion which is still utterly heretical in the US today (Miller 1986). Psychiatrists and other alcohol and drug treatment professionals throughout Europe also generally eschew the disease concept of alcoholism and, following the British Journal of Addiction and the World Health Organization, talk about 'alcohol dependence' (Edwards and Lader 1990).

Table 2.1 combines data from three sources to produce a profile of consumption patterns and AA membership in 24 Western nations. The total consumption of absolute (pure) alcohol for 1974 and 1984, along with the percentage of distilled spirits consumed for those two years, are the consumption figures of most relevance for the issues raised by this chapter. The percentages of pure alcohol in wine and beer are also listed for 1974 (they were not available for 1984). The temperance cultures are indicated by asterisks.

In the far right hand column the table shows the number of AA groups per million persons as computed by Mäkelä (1990). Since there is no formal membership in AA, all membership figures should be taken as rough approximations.

Most of the non-temperance cultures show negligible AA activity. This includes: France, Spain, Portugal, Austria, Italy, Hungary, Czechoslovakia, the Soviet Union, Denmark, and Poland. AA activity is also not very high in the temperance cultures of Sweden and Norway; Miller (1986) discusses some of the reasons for that.

Ireland and the Netherlands, both non-temperance countries, have a relatively high number of AA groups per million. Each one deserves special study as the story of the growth and spread of AA in each place is probably different.[2] Ireland has the highest rate of groups per million of any Western non-temperance culture. This may be due to several factors especially the impact in the early twentieth century of the Irish Protestant temperance tradition, and, perhaps, the influence of Irish-Americans who by all accounts seem to be the American Catholics most involved in AA in the US.

Germany, Switzerland, and Belgium are the remaining non-temperance cultures with some AA activity. Here too, each situation deserves study. Germany and Belgium have large numbers of military and corporate personnel from other temperance cultures, especially from the US, Canada, and the UK. That certainly accounts for some of the membership, perhaps for a lot of it. Switzerland (like Germany) has always had a small but steady temperance activity and AA membership there is in accord with that

---

[2] Mäkelä, in a personal communication, points out that perhaps the Netherlands should be grouped with the temperance cultures because of its relatively influential twentieth century temperance movement (de Lint 1981). Holland was also spirit-drinking and predominately Protestant. It is certainly the closest borderline case. Its high AA activity is therefore at least partially consistent with its relatively strong temperance tradition.

pattern. The hypotheses drawn from this chapter would suggest that native German and Swiss AA participation draws heavily, or primarily, from Protestants. Some evidence for that is also suggested by the case of Austria, an overwhelmingly Catholic country, with the same language as Germany and much of Switzerland; but Austria reports no AA groups at all.

The number of AA groups per million is a useful way of making some rough comparisons, but it distorts the general pattern of AA membership in the West. If we use the actual membership figures that Mäkelä presents we get a rather different picture.

There are about 781 700 AA members in all of the Western societies; 719 200 of them are in the temperance cultures — about 92 per cent. Of the temperance cultures, 704 845 are in English-speaking cultures — about 90 per cent. In the West, AA remains overwhelmingly a movement of the US, Canada, UK, and Australia. Indeed AA membership in the US and Canada totals 655 700 or 83.8 per cent of all AA membership in the West. And the US alone accounts for 585 800 persons or about 75 per cent of all AA membership in the West.

This general pattern of overall AA membership — predominately American, and overwhelmingly from other English-speaking cultures and some Nordic cultures — is in accord with the general argument of this chapter, and with the last one hundred and fifty years of temperance activity in the West.[3]

CONCLUSION

Prediction in the alcohol field is a tricky business and, as Griffith Edwards has suggested, is therefore usually best left to people with head scarfs and crystal balls. However, both Durkheim and Weber argued that all modern societies would become more like the Protestant cultures they had studied and would develop a heightened sense of individual autonomy and responsibility. It does not seem to be going out on too long a limb to suggest

---

[3] This chapter has focused on European and other Western societies because the classic temperance movements were Western movements, and because those societies share some broad cultural, economic, and political characteristics. Outside of the Western societies, AA activity is very limited. There is very little AA activity in either Africa or Asia. Mäkelä reports 5611 AA members in all of Africa, and 6570 in Asia. That means that Finland, with 9000 AA members has, by itself, more than either continent. And Australia, with 17 000 members has more than both continents combined.

The one place in the world where AA has apparently taken hold recently is in parts of Latin America, mainly in Mexico, and in some Central American, and Caribbean countries. Certainly people from the US, (and probably also from Protestant evangelical groups) have played some important roles in stimulating AA in Mexico and Central America (as they did, for example, in Sweden). Some of this activity is being researched by an international group (the International Collaborative Study of Alcoholics Anonymous); this study should form a fascinating part of the story of the diffusion of temperance ideas and of concern about alcohol problems.

that, as in the nineteenth century, Americans will to some extent successfully spread their conceptions and organizations to other societies; and that there will be in Europe some tendency toward what might be termed the 'Americanization' of alcohol issues. As a result, AA membership will likely grow in many countries over the next few decades. In the last few years, AA membership is reported to have increased substantially in Poland. However, it remains to be seen whether in Poland that process will continue and become institutionalized, or whether, like Father Mathew's crusade in the nineteenth century, it will peak and then fade.

Despite all the modernizing and homogenizing tendencies, it is likely that among Western countries the overall distribution and pattern of AA membership won't change very much in the next few decades. In the West, AA will remain primarily a temperance culture phenomenon, and more generally a Protestant one. Indeed, it does not seem likely that neo-temperance organizations or campaigns, stressing the dangerous character of alcohol, will find anywhere near the receptivity or popularity in *most* non-temperance Western cultures that they have found in the English-speaking and Nordic temperance cultures. It is unthinkable, for example, that any of the Mediterranean wine-drinking cultures would adopt measures like that of New York City and other localities which require any establishment selling beer, wine or spirits to display a sign warning pregnant women not to drink any alcoholic beverages. Mothers Against Drunk Drivers and Adult Children of Alcoholics will likewise never find much appeal in the non-temperance wine-drinking or beer-drinking societies (nor perhaps anywhere outside of the US).

This is not to say that 'objectively' non-temperance cultures will not experience relatively high levels of measurable 'alcohol problems'. Rather, the arguments presented in this chapter suggest that in the first third of the twenty-first century, as in the last third of the twentieth, the temperance cultures will continue to be the Western societies most interested in and concerned about alcohol problems. And that fact (or paradox) will remain (at least for some of us) a fascinating one to explore.[4]

[4] Some of the general findings of this chapter are in accord with the results of an interesting and innovative study by Simpura *et al.* (1990). The study involved asking people in Finland, Denmark, and West Germany to complete stories of everyday life. Many stories mentioned alcohol. The authors summarize their findings this way:

'On the surface, the material of this study seemed to repeat the stereotypical images of hedonistic Danes, heavy-drinking Finns, and ritualistic Germans. Going deeper it seemed that drinking has greatest expressive power in Finland, where references to drinking are more frequent and they are used effectively as social markers in the process of events described. In Denmark and Germany, drinking is more self-evident and is less remarkably used as a carrier of specific cultural meanings.'

This is what we would expect to find as the differences between a temperance culture and two non-temperance cultures.

ACKNOWLEDGEMENTS

This paper has benefited greatly from the advice of Robin Room, Craig Reinarman, Lillian Rubin, Laurie Phillips, Klaus Mäkelä, Griffith Edwards, and Basil Browne.

REFERENCES

Aries, P. (1962). *Centuries of childhood*. Random House, New York.

Alasuutari, P. (1990). Desire and craving: studies in a Cultural Theory of Alcoholism. Ph.d dissertation. University of Tampere, Finland.

Alcoholics Anonymous (1955). *Alcoholics Anonymous: the story of how many thousands of men and women have recovered from alcoholism* (2nd revised edn). Alcoholics Anonymous Publishing, New York.

Bengtsson, H. (1938). The temperance movement and temperance legislation in Sweden. *The Annals of the American Academy of Political and Social Science*, **197**.

Berridge, V. (1984). Editorial. *The British Journal of Addiction Centenary Edition, 1884–1984*, **79**, 1–6.

Blocker, J. S. (1989). *American temperance movements: cycles of reform*. Twayne, Boston.

Bruun, K. (1971). Finland: the non-medical approach. In Kiloh, L. G. and Bell, D. S (eds) *Alcoholism and drug dependence: 29th International Congress*, pp. 545–59. Butterworths, Sydney.

Cherrington, E. H. (ed.) (1924–1930). *Standard encyclopedia of the alcohol problem* (six volumes). American Issue Press, Westerville, Ohio.

Denzin, N. (1987). *The recovering alcoholic*. Sage, Newbury Park, California.

Durkheim, E. (1951). *Suicide*. Free Press, New York.

de Lint, J. (1981). Anti-drink propaganda and alcohol control measures: a report on the Dutch experiences. In Single, E. *et al.* (eds) *Alcohol, society and the state: 2 the social history of control policy in seven countries*, pp. 87–102. Addiction Research Foundation, Toronto.

Edwards, G. and Lader, M. (eds) (1990). *The nature of drug dependence*. Oxford University Press, Oxford.

Eliany, M. (1989). *Alcohol in Canada*. Minister of Supply and Services. Toronto, Canada.

Elias, N. (1978). *The history of manners: the civilizing process*, Vol. 1. Pantheon, New York.

Elias, N. (1982). *Power and civility: civilizing process*, Vol. 2. Pantheon, New York.

Epstein, B. L. (1980). *The politics of domesticity*. Wesleyan University Press, Middletown, Connecticut.

Eriksen, S. (1990). Drunken Danes and sober Swedes? Religious revivalism and the Temperance Movements as keys to Danish and Swedish folk cultures. In Strath, B. (ed.) *Language and the construction of class identities: the struggle*

for discursive power in social organization, Scandinavia and Germany after 1800. Department of History, Gottenburg (book page proofs).
Falk P. and Sulkunen, P. (1983). Drinking on the screen: an analysis of a mythical male fantasy in Finnish films. *Social Science Information* **22**, 387-410.
Foucault, M. (1965). *Madness and civilization.* Pantheon, New York.
Foucault, M. (1977). *Discipline and punishment: The birth of the prison.* Pantheon, New York.
Foucault, M. (1978). *The history of sexuality*, Vol. 1. Pantheon, New York.
Freud, S. (1961). *Civilization and its discontents.* Norton, New York.
Geertz, C. (1973). *The interpretation of cultures.* Basic Books, New York.
Greven, P. (1977) *The Protestant temperament.* Knopf, New York.
Gusfield, J. R. (1986). *Symbolic crusade: status politics and the American Temperance Movement* (2nd edn). University of Illinois Press, Urbana.
Frykman, J. and Lofgren, O. (1987). *Culture builders: a historical anthropology of middle class life* (trans. A. Crozier). Rutgers University Press, New Brunswick and London.
Harrison, B. (1971). *Drink and the Victorians.* University of Pittsburg Press, Pittsburg Pennsylvania.
Hudson, W. (1961). *American Protestantism.* University of Chicago Press, Chicago.
Keller, M. and Guridi, C. (1976). *Statistics on consumption of alcohol and on alcoholism.* Rutgers Center for Alcohol Studies and *The Journal of Studies on Alcohol.* New Brunswick, New Jersey.
Kerr, K. A. (1985). *Organized for prohibition: a new history of the Anti-Saloon League.* Yale University Press, New Haven.
Kurtz, E. (1979). *Not God: a history of Alcoholics Anonymous.* Hazelden, Center City Minnesota.
Leach, B. and Norris, J. L. (1977). Factors in the development of Alcoholics Anonymous. In Kissen, B. and Begleiter, H. (eds) *The Treatment and Rehabilitation of the Chronic Alcoholic* (Vol. 5 of *The Biology of Alcoholism*), pp. 441-541. Plenum Press, New York.
Lender, M. E. (1984). *Dictionary of American temperance biography: from temperance reform to alcohol research.* Greenwood, Westport, Connecticut.
Lender, M. E. and Karnchanapee, K. R. (1977). Temperance tales: antiliquor fiction and American attitudes toward alcoholics in the late 19th and early 20th centuries. *Journal of Studies on Alcohol*, **38**, 1347-70.
Levine, H. G. (1978). The discovery of addiction: changing conceptions of habitual drunkenness in America. *Journal of Studies on Alcohol*, **39**, 143-74.
Levine, H. G. (1980). Women and temperance in nineteenth century America. In O. Kalant (ed.) *Research advances in alcohol and drug problems*, Vol. 5. Plenum, New York.
Levine, H. G. (1983). The good creature of god and the demon rum: colonial and 19th century American ideas about alcohol, accidents and crime. In R. Room and G. Collins (eds) *Alcohol and disinhibition*, Research Monograph No. 12, pp. 111-61. US National Institute on Alcohol Abuse and Alcoholism, Washington. DC.
Levine, H. G. (1984). The alcohol problem in America: from temperance to alcoholism. *British Journal of Addiction*, **79**, 109-19.

Lolli, G., Serianni, E., Golder, G. M., and Luzzatto-Fegiz, P. (1958). *Alcohol in Italian Culture*. Yale Center of Alcohol Studies, New Haven.

MacAndrew, C. and Edgerton, R. (1969). *Drunken comportment: a societal explanation*. Aldine, Chicago.

Malcolm, E. (1986). *'Ireland free, Ireland sober': drink and temperance in nineteenth century Ireland*. Gill and MacMillan, Dublin.

Mäkelä, K. (1990). Social and cultural preconditions of AA and factors associated with the strength of AA. Presented at the 16th Annual Meetings of the Kettil Bruun Society for Social and Epidemiological Research on Alcohol, Budapest, June.

Miller, W. R. (1986). Haunted by the *Zeitgeist*: reflections on contrasting treatment goals and concepts of alcoholism in Europe and the United States. In T. Babor (ed.) *Alcohol and culture*, pp. 110–29. New York Academy of Medicine, New York.

Mills, C. W. (1959). *The sociological imagination*. Oxford, New York.

Nordic Voices (1984). special issue of *Daedalus* Spring.

Partanen, J. (1987). Serious drinking, serious alcohol policy: the case of the Soviet Union. *Contemporary Drug Problems*, Winter, pp. 507–38.

Paulson, R. E. (1973). *Women's suffrage and prohibition*. Scott, Foresman, Glenview, Illinois.

Prestwich, P. E. (1988). *Drink and the politics of social reform: Antialcoholism in France since 1870*. Society for the Promotion of Science and Scholarship, Palo Alto, California.

Reinarman, C. (1988). The social construction of an alcohol problem: the case of Mothers Against Drunk Driving and social control in the 1980s. *Theory and Society*, **17**, 91–119.

Roberts, J. (1984). *Drink, temperance and the working class in Nineteenth-Century Germany*. George Allen and Unwin, Boston.

Room R. (1984). A 'reverence for strong drink': the lost generation and the elevation of alcohol in American culture. *Journal of Studies on Alcohol*, **45**, 540–6.

Room, R. (1989). Responses to alcohol-related problems in an international perspective: characterizing and explaining cultural wetness and dryness. Presented at an International Conference in Santo Stefano Belbo, Italy. Available from the Alcohol Research Group, Berkeley, California.

Room, R. (1990). The Impossible dream? Routes to reducing alcohol problems in a temperance culture. Presented at Nordic Council for Alcohol and Drug Research Conference on Alcohol Policy and Social Change, Hveragerdi, Iceland, 3–7 September.

Room, R. G. W. (1988). The dialectic of drinking in Australian life: from the run corps to the wine column. *Australian Drug and Alcohol Review*, **7**, 413–37.

Room R. and Collins G. (eds) (1983). *Alcohol and disinhibition*, Research Monograph No. 12, US National Institute on Alcohol Abuse and Alcoholism, Washington, DC.

Rorabaugh, W. J. (1979). *The alcoholic republic*. Oxford University Press, New York.

Sadoun, R., Lolli, G. and Silverman, M. (1965). *Drinking in French culture*. Rutgers Center for Alcohol, New Brunswick, New Jersey.

Simpura, J. (ed.) (1987). *Finnish drinking habits*. Finnish Foundation for Alcohol Studies, Helsinki.

Simpura, J., Fahrenkrug, H., Hyttinen, M., and Thorsen, T. (1990). Drinking, everyday life situations and cultural norms in Denmark, Finland, and West Germany: an experiment with nonactive role-playing. *Journal of Drug Issues*, 20, 403–16.

Smith, R. E. F. and Christian, D. (1984). *Bread and salt: a social and economic history of food and drink in Russia*. Cambridge University Press, London.

Sulkunen, I. (1986). *Temperance as civic religion: the Temperance Movement and Popular Organization in Finland from the 1870's to the years after the Great Strike of 1905*. Currently being translated for the Finnish Foundation for Alcohol Studies, Helsinki.

Thompson, W. (1935). *The control of liquor in Sweden*. Columbia University Press, New York.

Tyrell, I. (1979). *Sobering up: from temperance to prohibition in antebellum America, 1800–1860*. Greenwood, Westport, Connecticut.

Vogt, I. (1981). Cultural beliefs and government propensities to control or ignore drinking problems: a historical comparison of Germany and the U.S. In *The Drinking and Drug Practices Surveyor*, # **17** pp. 4–8.

Weber, M. (1958). *The Protestant ethic and the spirit of capitalism* (trans. T. Parsons). Scribners, New York.

Weber, M. (1963). *The sociology of religion*. Beacon, Boston.

Wuorinen, J. H. (1931). *The prohibition experiment in Finland*. Columbia University Press, New York.

3

Correlation and causality: notes on epistemological problems in substance abuse research

OLE-JØRGEN SKOG

INTRODUCTION

In an intuitive understanding of causality, a cause is something that produces or brings about an effect. We will here treat 'causality' as a primitive concept, and it is doubtful that the concept can be analytically reduced to even more primitive concepts, that do not themselves presuppose an understanding of causality. The author has never seen such an analysis, and shares Anscombe's doubt that it is possible to make one (Anscombe 1975).

Our topic is instead how we know that a certain relation is a causal relation. What are the criteria that allow us to assert that C is a cause of E, and to distinguish causal relations from non-causal relations? And what are the limits of causal explanations — can everything be explained causally?

The text is organized as follows. The first sections discuss some of the main philosophical theories of causality. We start by reviewing Hume's position, and argue that Hume's criteria are defective for at least three different reasons. The third section briefly discusses definitions of causality in terms of necessary and sufficient conditions and in terms of counterfactual conditionals. All are defective in one way or another. We argue that the actionist view is the only one that adequately deals with the fundamental problem of causal inference, and that fits the methodology experimental scientists actually use to identify causes.

After this general introduction, causal inference is discussed at a more practical level. The fourth section studies the strengths and limitations of experimental methods, with particular reference to some basic questions in substance abuse research. The case is argued that although experiments may provide answers to many important issues, several questions are left unaccounted for by this methodology. The fifth section, discusses Suppes' probabilistic theory of causality and its application to non-experimental methods, arguing that some of the standard problems in non-experimental research can be overcome by better theories and by methodological pluralism. The sixth section raises the question of whether everything has a cause (determinism), and discusses some consequences for empirical research if a negative answer to this question is presumed.

HUME'S CRITERION OF CONSTANT CONJUNCTION

According to Hume, the essential elements of the idea of causation are the three empirical relations contiguity, succession, and constant conjunction. 'Beyond these three circumstances of contiguity, priority, and constant conjunction, I can discover nothing in this cause...' (Hume in *An Abstract Treatise of Human Nature*, quoted after Beauchamp and Rosenberg 1981, p. 4). Necessary connection, according to Hume, is a mental idea, acquired by habit, so that the idea of the one determines the mind to form the idea of the other.

Hume's exact definition of causality reads as follows (quoted after Beauchamp and Rosenberg 1981, p. 5): we may define a cause to be 'an object precedent and contiguous to another, and where all the objects resembling the former are placed in like relations of precedency and contiguity to those objects, that resemble the latter'.

Hume's conception is not entirely satisfactory, however. Three problems will briefly be discussed, all of which are tied in with Hume's criterion of constant conjunction. There are two practical problems with this criterion, and one problem of a more fundamental nature. Let me start with the practical problems.

The problem of similarity

While in many types of causal systems similar causes produce similar effects, this is not always true. An important class of phenomena where this is not true is studied in the new discipline called chaos theory. Chaos theory is concerned with complex systems that are non-linear (in the mathematical sense), and it turns out that such systems may be fundamentally different from linear systems. Although completely deterministic, such systems may behave in a quite irregular way, resembling a stochastic, rather than a deterministic process. Of particular interest in the present context is the fact that two identical systems, differing only infinitesimally in their starting values, may rapidly diverge and become very different after a short time. Hence, however precise our knowledge of the system at some state, it will be impossible to predict its future course of development. Meteorological systems exemplify this kind of phenomena. In certain cases forecasts are impossible, because minutely small variations in the parameters of the system (well below the measurement errors) produce substantially different outcomes (cf. Palmer 1989). It is important to realize that no random mechanism is involved in this case.

A related type of unpredictability is called bifurcation. In non-linear systems, when the parameters of the system are changed gradually, the state of the system may change smoothly up to a certain point. Beyond that point, however, two possible states occur, and which one is 'chosen' may be essentially unpredictable. An example of such a system is the perfect ferromagnet. Beyond a certain temperature, the so-called Curie temperature, there is no ferromagnetism. The spins of the electrons are essentially uncorrelated, except over very short distances — too short to create the large-scale pattern which is responsible for ferromagnetism. As the item is gradually cooled, small-scale order increases but there is no qualitative change. However, at the Curie temperature, large-scale order occurs abruptly, and the item spontaneously becomes ferromagnetic. Spins line up over infinitely large distances, as the temperature drops below the Curie temperature. However, it is impossible to predict the direction of the magnet in advance (Wilson 1979). Very small perturbations in the system's state above the Curie temperature may produce very different results below the Curie temperature.

In both of these examples, Hume's similarity criterion — considered as a practical empirical rule — breaks down. Very similar causes may fail to produce similar effects, although the underlying mechanism is indeed causal. Hence, in some cases similarity is not enough — nothing less than identity will suffice.

The problem of constancy

In some cases it may not be necessary for a scientist to make repeated observations in order to conclude that a causal relationship exists. For instance, assume that a biologist has created a particular mutation of a primitive organism. He has only one individual and it is extremely unlikely that he will be able to produce another. The organism is green. For some strange reason — which need not concern us here — he suspects that the organism will immediately and permanently become red if it is exposed to alcohol. He may then test his hypothesis simply by exposing it to alcohol. If it turns red, he will conclude that his hypothesis was right, and that alcohol actually caused this change. How does he know that the change was not caused by some other factor that the organism was exposed to, and how does he know that the temporal correlation of the two events (exposure to alcohol and change in colour) was not a coincidence? Since he is a trained experimental scientist he anticipated this question, and had designed a sophisticated set-up, controlling every possible factor that the organism was exposed to, and randomizing the time of the exposition to alcohol. Thus, there was an exceedingly small likelihood that the organism should change its colour by chance at the exact moment when alcohol was applied to it.

Although this example may not satisfy the philosopher, it should be good enough for empirical scientists, who cannot afford to make the best the enemy of the good. We can never be *perfectly* sure that our procedures are good enough. If perfection was the standard, then there would be no empirical science at all.

In any case, bringing in more organisms — if this were possible after all — would not qualitatively change the situation. We could reduce the likelihood of a coincidence even further, but this would only be a change in degree, and not a qualitative change. Secondly, we could not be perfectly sure that all specimens were in fact identical or similar enough to count as replicas of each other. In the light of the first argument above one must be open to the possibility that even the slightest difference in genetical make-up could make a significant difference.

Many phenomena, particularly socio-historical phenomena, may not occur more than once. Alternatively, repeated occurrences may not be similar enough for them to count as replications of each other. Hence, if one insists that constant conjunction is an absolute requirement as a criterion for causality, one is simply saying that causality is not a relevant epistemological category in social science. The author is not willing to draw that conclusion.

Both the problem of similarity and the problem of constancy are practical problems, encountered when we apply Hume's theoretical criteria in our daily work as empirical scientists. They do not represent serious threats to Hume's conceptualization (or theoretical definition) of causality. However, the third problem is conceptual, rather than practical.

The problem of spuriousness

The basic flaw in Hume's conception of causality is that his criteria fails to distinguish between true causal relationships and epiphenomena or spurious correlations. If two phenomena are both products of the same cause, they will constantly occur together, but there is no causal relation between them. This is the problem that many empirical life sciences constantly face — namely to find out whether a phenomenon that tends to occur together with another, is actually the cause of the other, or whether there is a third factor that produces both of them.

Beauchamp and Rosenberg's defence of Hume cites two Humean criteria for separating accidental and causal regularities. The first is *inductive support* — that testing a number of instances under a variety of circumstances, produces degrees of evidence and instills further confidence that generalizations really are law-like, and not spurious. The second criterion is called predictive confidence — the *confidence* people place in factual evidence. By this is probably meant the strength of the mental idea, acquired by habit, but also theoretical support from other causal generalizations, as well as failure to see mechanisms that could have produced a spurious relationship.

Variation of circumstances is not necessarily a good criterion — a spurious correlation may be quite persistent across circumstances. Moreover, the first argument above indicates that the causal relation sometimes may be very sensitive to changes in circumstances. The cause C may have effect E, only under very specific circumstances, and changes in circumstances may sometimes produce qualitatively new results. Hence, with this criterion there is a risk of throwing out the baby with the bath water.

Confidence is a criterion of significant heuristic value in empirical science. Sometimes we simply do not have much more to offer as 'proof' for a causal hypothesis, than consistency with the remaining body of knowledge, and failure to see realistic alternative explanations. On other occasions, however, we are in fact able to reach beyond this criterion, and this is the kind of situation we shall now analyse somewhat more closely.

NECESSITY, COUNTERFACTUALS, AND EXPERIMENTAL DESIGNS

At this point, it will be useful to briefly summarize another branch of causal theory, namely the analysis of causality in terms of necessary and sufficient conditions, that frequently occurs in many philosophical texts.

Unconditionally, a cause C (the red billiard ball hitting the white) is neither necessary nor sufficient for its effect E (the white billiard ball going into the pocket). The cause is not sufficient since the effect may be prevented by another event (say, by someone stopping the white ball), and it is not necessary since some other event (say, an earthquake) could have produced the same effect. In both cases, other factors are operating. Hence, at the very least one has to assume that everything else remains unchanged, in order to analyse the causal relation in terms of necessary and sufficient conditions.

Some scholars have defined the cause C as a *ceteris paribus* sufficient condition for E. Given the circumstances, the effect E *must* occur when the cause C has already occurred. Hence, if the effect has *not* occurred, then the cause cannot have occurred either. Others have defined the cause as a *ceteris paribus* necessary condition. Given the circumstances, if the cause had *not* occurred, then neither would the effect. Both definitions run into problems.

The necessary condition

Consider a spurious relation, where C and E are both products of some common cause A, and that under the circumstances considered, E can only be produced by A. (In effect, A is sufficient to produce C, and both sufficient and necessary for E to occur). The situation may be schematically represented as follows:

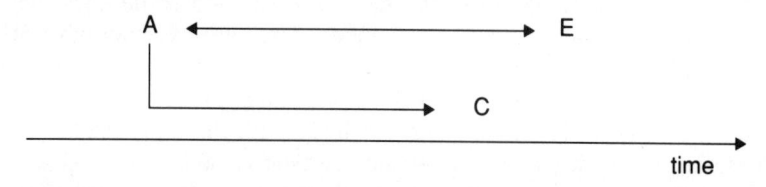

```
         A ←─────────────────→ E
         │
         └─────────────→ C
   ─────────────────────────────────→
                                  time
```

Now, if C has not occurred, then neither can A have occurred, since A would have produced C. But when A has not occurred, it cannot have produced E. Hence E is also absent, since nothing else could produce it. Therefore, C is *ceteris paribus* necessary for E. Since C is not the cause of E, however, the criterion clearly does not help us to separate causal from spurious relations.

The sufficient condition

It may be true that both C and E have occurred, and also that C is *ceteris paribus* sufficient for E. Nevertheless, C may not be the true cause of E. The counter argument is analogue to the previous one. Suppose that A produces both C and E, and also that A is the only way that C can be brought about, under the circumstances considered, i.e. we have the following situation:

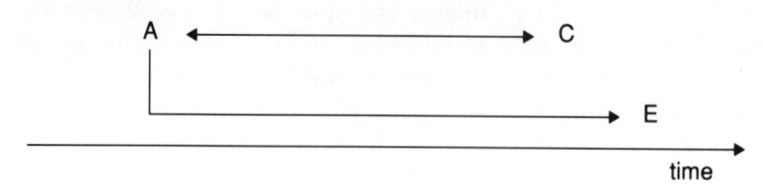

```
         A ←─────────────────→ C
         │
         └─────────────→ E
   ─────────────────────────────────→
                                  time
```

If C has occurred, this is because A has occurred, and A will secure that E occurs. If the effect E has not occurred, neither can A have occurred (since it would have produced E, if it had), and when A is absent, C cannot have occurred (since, by assumption, nothing else could have produced it).

In spite of these difficulties, the counterfactual hypothesis has remained a significant part of intuitive ideas on causality: *Ceteris paribus*, if the cause had not occurred, then neither would the effect have occurred. However, the solution to this dilemma is not to be found by a formal logical analysis, of the type frequently found in philosophical texts on causality, but by asking how scientists can and actually do get around the problem of spuriousness.

Before addressing that issue, let me briefly outline the counterfactual analysis in terms of the concept of alternative worlds (Lewis 1973; Glymour 1986). Imagine a collection of possible worlds, and that it is meaningful to compare possible worlds in terms of closeness or similarity to the actual world. Then the counterfactual definition of cause can be stated as follows (Glymour 1986, p. 965):

X causes Y if and only if X is true in the actual world and Y is true in the actual world and in the closest (to the actual world) possible world in which X is not true, Y is not true.

The criterion of being closest is introduced since in a very different world where X does not obtain, Y may be brought about by something else.

Unfortunately, this definition does not really get around the problem of spurious correlation, for the same reason as the sufficiency and necessity conditions fail: assume that A produces both C and E. In the closest alternative world, the factor A that produces the apparent cause (as well as the effect) will not obtain, and the effect will not occur either. Hence, even spurious correlations fulfil the criterion.

The concept of alternative worlds is still useful, however, since it comes close to describing what scientists actually do in controlled experiments. When a scientist wants to test whether giving a new medication (event C) cures a certain disease (event E), he choses two identical 'local worlds', applies C to patients in one local world, while patients in the other local world get an inactive placebo. Since the local worlds are presumed identical, any difference between the outcomes must be caused by C.

The fundamental problem of causal inference, as Holland (1986) has called it, is that it is impossible to observe simultaneously what happens to an entity (a system, a subject) both when it is exposed to and not exposed to a cause. Often, however, we have a group of subjects, some of which are exposed to C and some of which are not. If the subjects are selected to conditions C and not-C by some systematic mechanism, we run the risk that the mechanism will produce non-comparable groups, and that this will produce differences in outcome that are not the result of differences in treatment. In this case the selection mechanism creates spurious correlation between C and E since it systematically gives C to subjects who will display E and non-C to subjects who will display not-E. However, by randomizing subjects to treatment (C) and control (not-C), this difficulty is avoided, and the fundamental problem is solved. The randomization procedure secures that the groups are statistically 'identical', and the counterfactual is no longer contrary to fact.

From a philosophical point of view it is worth noting that the validity of this procedure depends on the experimenters ability to create statistically identical groups. Hence, we must presume that there is no unknown, godlike (or devilish) factor D that determines both the allocation of subjects and the outcome of the experiment. This presumption, which the author calls the action–theoretical postulate of experimental methodology, cannot in itself be proved by scientific methods — it is a metaphysical principle.

Although this type of experimental design is typically used and described in situations with multiple subjects, it seems to the author that the fundamental logic of the approach does not require more than one subject. This was illustrated in our previous example with the mutant organism with alcohol allergy. By observing the organism over a long series of time intervals without C, then applying C at a randomly chosen interval and observing it for another long series of time intervals, we have essentially obtained the same thing. Subjects are replaced by time intervals as units of observation. Which units get what treatment is determined by a random mechanism in both cases. There is one fundamental difference, however, and this is that there exists a natural ordering of time intervals, while no such ordering exists for the subjects. The ordering of time intervals has the consequence that the units are not independent in terms of what 'treatment' they get. However, statistical methods for dealing with this complication are now available (cf. Box and Jenkins 1976), and as long as the administration of C is randomized, no difference of fundamental importance can be seen between the two approaches.

The essence of the experimental strategy consists in actively preventing spuriousness, that is, preventing that whatever produces C, also produces E. Action on behalf of the scientist is required, and philosophically we leave the classical Humean domain of causal theory, which is purely observational, and enter the actionist domain suggested by von Wright (1971) and others. To experiment, means to manipulate the world in a systematic way.

The actionist analysis of causality has been charged with anthropomorphism. For instance, it is claimed that the analysis precludes a causal relation between events for which no manipulative techniques are available, or that the analysis precludes causal relations independent of human actions of any kind (Beauchamp and Rosenberg 1981, p. 206). If the actionist approach is seen as an attempt to define what causality 'really is', this objection is understandable. However, this is not the case. The idea is to improve on Hume's criteria, and find an empirical criterion that helps us to distinguish between causal relations and spurious relations. The action-theoretical analysis does not tie causation *as such* to human action — causation is not mind-dependent or action-dependent. However, *learning* about causation is mind-dependent, and — according to action theory — it can be action-dependent. In short, actionist or experimental criteria address epistemological problems, not ontological ones.

THE STRENGTH AND LIMITATIONS OF EXPERIMENTAL DESIGNS

It is thus necessary to make controlled experiments in order to unambiguously conclude that a correlation is signifying that C has produced E, rather than that C and E tend to occur together for some other reason.

Fortunately, many important research questions about substance abuse can be addressed by experimental methods. This is so both at the biomedical or molecular level, at the psychological level or the level of individual organisms, as well as at the aggregate level of socio-cultural groups or societies. Although the availability of the experimental method clearly decreases as we move towards higher levels, even the effects of aggregate changes in availability of alcohol have been studied by way of controlled experimental methods.

Unfortunately, however, the experimental method does not automatically and straightforwardly allow causal conclusions, particularly not at the level of the individual or groups of individuals. When we study human behaviour we encounter problems that are not present at lower levels.

Consider the following example: we want to see whether a sleeping pill works, and give it to some test subjects, while control subjects receive an inactive placebo. A double blind design is used. Assume that we find no difference between the groups. Are we allowed to conclude that our pill has no effect? Not necessarily. Assume that all, or most, of our subjects often have problems falling asleep, but know from prior experience that sleeping pills normally solve their problem. Now, our subjects often cannot fall asleep, simply because they are afraid that they will not fall asleep — a self-fulfilling expectation, as it were. By taking the pill they do not have to worry, since they know from past experience that they will fall asleep in less than 30 min, due to the pharmacological effects of the pill. Relieved of their worries, they fall asleep immediately — before any pharmacological effects have occurred. This so-called non-standard causal chain should work for both groups, and thus we may not find a difference between placebo and the pill, even though there actually is a significant pharmacological difference.

The problem in this case is due to the fact that our subjects have prior experience. This can be avoided in many pharmacological experiments, but it is not easy to avoid this problem in the case of alcohol. In order to get around this particular problem, Alan Marlatt developed the so-called balanced placebo design, where not only the substance delivered to the subjects is manipulated, but also their beliefs about what they get. Hence, in this design there are four distinct experimental conditions, compared to only two in the conventional double blind placebo design:

Subjects receive	Subjects believe
Alcohol	Alcohol
	Placebo
Placebo	Alcohol
	Placebo

Numerous experiments have been made with this methodology, in an attempt to separate the pharmacological and the psychological effects of alcohol, and the interaction between them. The behavioural dimensions studied include loss-of-control, destructive and aggressive behaviour, sexual behaviour, fear and anxiety etc. Undoubtedly, these experiments have shed considerable light on these issues, and the results have very often underlined the significance of psychological factors, including set, setting, prior learning, cultural myths etc.

Some writers have even concluded, on the basis of the results, that pharmacological effects are causally irrelevant in relation to these behavioural dimensions. Such conclusions are not warranted, however, and their proponents clearly go beyond the limits of the design. It should not be forgotten that, in these experiments very small amounts of alcohol are used, to prevent the subjects disclosing the design. Hence, according to the ordinary rules of scientific inference, one is not allowed to draw conclusions about the relative effects of pharmacology and psychology when it comes to large amounts of alcohol. In particular, one is not allowed to conclude that the pharmacological effects of large amounts of alcohol are irrelevant in relation to, say, loss-of-control and aggressive behaviour.

What these experiments actually demonstrate, is that psychological effects are quite important, and that pharmacological mechanisms are not linked to behaviour by simple and direct mechanical processes. However, they do not prove that pharmacological effects are irrelevant. In fact, the design is really not very well suited for uncovering the 'true' pharmacological effects of alcohol. If one finds an alcohol effect in these experiments, one must always be open to the possibility that the subjects — either consciously or sub-consciously — have disclosed the true content of their drink, and have reacted according to their psychological expectations. Hence, any pharmacological effect may be dismissed by those who remain sceptical about any specific type of pharmacological effect. But this simply amounts to saying that the design cannot uncover pharmacological effects, if they should exist after all.

The lesson to be learned from this, I think, is that not everything can easily be manipulated. Hence, the experimental method has its limitations — it will not answer all our questions.

Let us next consider a related problem. Normally, when we make experimental manipulations, we have definite causal mechanisms in mind, that we wish to test. However, our manipulations are seldom perfectly precise, and they normally have several aspects or by-products that are not really intended. The so-called Hawthorne effect exemplifies this problem, and it may very well have relevance in relation to substance abuse. Consider the following example: a group of treatment workers have developed some new ideas about treatment of alcohol abusers, and wish to test their method against conventional techniques. Suppose they use the most sophisticated experimental methods, randomizing patients etc., and suppose that independent researchers find that the new method gives better outcomes. Does this prove their hypothesis? Not necessarily. It may very well be the case that the superior result was simply a product of greater enthusiasm among treatment personnel for the new method (say because it is a *new* method, or because it is *their* method), rather than any intrinsic attribute of the new treatment. Or the abusers may have improved because they received more attention and a different type of attention, compared to the usual state of affairs. In either case, the superior outcome may be a transient effect, and may disappear when the method is no longer 'new'.

Treatment research also presents us with another causal inference problem. The results of controlled experimental comparisons of treatment and no-treatment (or minimal intervention) have been rather disappointing for those who like to believe that it is possible to help people with a drinking problem. Does this mean that treatment has no, or only marginal effects? Or are there some (possibly indirect) effects that escape conventional methods?

Let us — for the sake of the argument — look at the following scenario: a person recognizes that he has a substance abuse problem, and he has decided that he needs treatment for his abuse. Now, it can be imagined that the important causal mechanisms are embedded in this initial part of the process, and that it is more or less irrelevant for his prognosis whether or not he actually receives treatment, and what kind of treatment he gets. If this were the case we would expect to find no difference between the treatment and the no-treatment group in an experimental design with randomization etc. It could still be argued that treatment has an effect, however, since our subject's recognition of his problem may depend on the very fact that there are treatment institutions. If there had been no such institutions, he might have continued his alcohol abuse until, say, succumbing in liver coma. The presence of treatment institutions may have such effects, partly because they are parts of the social conception of abuse as a problem, and partly by signalling a constructive hope that addicts can learn to control their problems.

In conclusion, the substance abuse researchers' task is not a simple one. As the examples illustrate, it can be quite difficult to find valid answers to causal questions, even if we use controlled experimental methods. The difficulties do not stop here, however.

So far, we have been concerned with what is sometimes called the *internal* validity of a design. In the social sciences, we often encounter problems of another sort. The *external* validity of an experiment refers to the problem of drawing conclusions from observations made in a controlled situation, to real-life situations. Control means changing, and we may run the risk of changing the conditions to such an extent that the result has little or no bearing on social reality. Hence, psychology and social science may sometimes face an unsolvable conflict between external and internal validity. If we do not experiment, we cannot decide which relations are spurious and which are not. And if we do experiment, we may learn a lot about 'artificial' societies, but little about real ones.

The solution to this conflict must be a pragmatic one — namely to use as many different methods and approaches as possible to shed light on the phenomenon of interest. Therefore, science needs both experimental and non-experimental methods. Each method has its weaknesses, but different methods suffer from different kinds of weaknesses, and by combining many different methods one can hope to establish results beyond reasonable doubt.

NON-EXPERIMENTAL METHODS

In many cases we cannot experiment, and in other cases we are not able to study each separate causal factor, keeping everything else the same. A concept of causality defined only in terms of *ceteris paribus* will not be very useful under such circumstances.

Suppes' (1970) probabilistic theory of causation deals with this kind of situation. Suppes starts by defining a prima facie cause of an event, as an event that temporally precedes it and that is positively associated with it. He then defines a spurious cause of an event as a prima facie cause of the effect that is, in fact, conditionally independent of the effect, given a second event that is temporally prior to the prima facie cause, and that is conditionally positively associated with the effect given the prima facie cause. A genuine cause is a prima facie cause that is not spurious. Somewhat simplified, this can be rephrased as saying that an association is causal if it cannot be entirely done away with by controlling for other factors.

The standard statistical approach is essentially an implementation of Suppes' theory, and amounts to recording all the variables ($D_1, D_2, \ldots$) we can think of, that could be causes of both C and E, and thus potentially produce a spurious correlation between C and E. By mathematical methods one can estimate whether a relationship remains after statistically controlling the impact of all these 'confounders'. The problems with this strategy are two-fold.

On the one hand one may easily throw out the baby with the bath water. If there is no relationship left between C and E after controlling for all the Ds, this may be because there is no causal relationship, or because there is too little variation left after controlling for confounders. The latter problem — so-called multicolinearity — occurs when there is a high (statistical) correlation between C and the Ds and this is very often the case in real life situations. For instance, in the 1940s it was claimed that vitamin deficiency, and not alcohol as such, caused cirrhosis of the liver. This claim was apparently based on the observation that the correlation between cirrhosis and alcohol disappeared once vitamin deficiency was controlled for, since in the data available at the time the people who had high alcohol intake also had vitamin deficiency.

Unfortunately, multicolinearity is a much ignored problem in substance abuse research. Very often statistical analyses are seen where this problem is not adequately dealt with, and the author strongly suspects that many negative results are spurious because of this.

The second problem with the so-called control variable approach, is that it may be difficult to find all relevant control variables. If some important factor is left out, i.e. if we have failed to take all relevant Ds into consideration, spurious correlation may prevail. In fact, sometimes — under very special circumstances — we may actually be worse off after having made the control, than when we started (cf. Lieberson 1985).

To fix ideas, consider the following example: a substantial correlation between the drinking habits of Norwegian parents and their adolescent children have been found, and it is also found that adolescents are more frequently intoxicated if they are given alcohol by their parents. These relationships survive statistical controls in a multivariate analysis (Pedersen 1990).

Is this a spurious correlation or a causal relationship? If the latter is the case, parents can reduce their children's drunkenness by not giving them alcohol. However, this is the kind of relationship which is very difficult to analyse with cross-sectional data, and one can easily imagine several mechanisms that would create this kind of correlation, and that would escape conventional statistical control. For instance, in wet and liberal strata of the population, both parents and children tend to drink much and the parents may tend to give their children alcohol. In dryer and more restrictive strata, both generations drink less and it is less likely that parents give alcohol to their children. Hence, a correlation would exist, but it does not follow that the children in the wet subculture would drink less if their parents stopped giving them alcohol. Moreover, in this case one can even imagine that the causal arrow is going in a direction opposite to the one suggested, since adolescents who seldom drink may seldom ask their parents for alcohol.

In cases such as this, where experimentation is impossible or at least very difficult, and where spuriousness due to selection bias is very likely, one can strengthen a causal hypothesis by bringing in other types of data. Aggregate level data may sometimes be quite useful for this purpose, since at the aggregate level, selection bias is typically not present to the same extent. For instance, the fact that the liver cirrhosis mortality rates covaries fairly closely with per capita alcohol consumption, both across countries and within each country over time, suggests that alcohol is in fact an important aetiological factor, and that individual level correlations between alcohol intake and cirrhosis is not spurious.

Sophisticated methods for analysing aggregate level data have become available in recent years. These methods reduce the risk for spurious correlation substantially (Skog 1988). Unfortunately, such methods are still not widely used, and it is surprising to see that researchers who use very sophisticated methods when they analyse individual level data, relapse to very crude and simplistic methods when it comes to aggregate data.

Of course, not even the most sophisticated analytical techniques can fully compensate for the fact that only non-experimental data are at hand. However, so-called quasi-experimental designs come very close to the 'real thing'. By taking advantage of naturally occurring rapid changes in the causal factor of interest, say the availability of alcohol, one may come very close to a real experimental design. Provided that the political event that caused the change in availability has not directly affected the effects the researcher is interested in, say the alcohol consumption level, alcohol problem rates etc., then causal inference should be reasonably safe under these circumstances. However, if the event is the product of a unique alcohol or drug political situation — it may perhaps be the result of strong public opinions on the matter — this presumption may not be valid.

Strikes at the retail level for alcoholic beverages have frequently been used as natural experiments, and in this case the key presumption is probably valid. Unfortunately, nothing in this world is free, and there is a snag. A strike is typically an unusual kind of situation, and it can be argued that the consumers react differently in an unusual situation. If for no other reason, consumers could react differently because they know that the strike will eventually come to an end. Hence, the old problem with external validity pops up again, since we cannot safely assume that the effects of the strike carry over to 'normal' changes in availability.

So far we have been discussing questions where experimental methods could have provided an answer, if practical problems had not prevented us from applying such methods. Typically, these questions are of the following type: 'Does C produce (cause) E?' For instance, does excessive drinking cause cirrhosis, does treatment help the client to reduce his drinking, do parents' giving alcohol to their children increase the children's drinking etc. In all of these cases, non-experimental methods are second-best solutions.

There is, however, another important class of causal questions where this is not the case. Suppose we ask why alcohol problems increased in Sweden in the late 1950s, or why alcohol consumption decreased strongly in Norway during the 1840s, or why Mr X stopped drinking in 1990? These are questions about historical events. They require causal explanations, but they cannot be answered by experimental methods. The first set of questions are of a general (some would say law-like) nature, while the latter are about particular historical events. Moreover, the first set focuses the cause and asks what kind of effect it produces, while the second focuses the effect and asks what its cause might be.

In order to be able to answer the second class of questions about particulars, we clearly need to have an understanding of general relationships. For instance, the decrease in alcohol consumption in Norway in the 1840s may — partly at least — be explained by noting that prices increased and availability decreased, and by using the general fact, established in other studies, that prices and availability tend to affect the consumption level in this way.

However, in situations such as this, we encounter a new problem. Assume that the effect E has occurred, and that C has also occurred and that we know generally that C causes E. Nevertheless we cannot be sure that C actually caused E in this particular case, since it may have been caused by another factor D, that also occurred. In this particular case, the effect E may have been causally over-determined, and D may have pre-empted C by producing E before C had the chance to operate.

More generally, in the real world, numerous causal factors operate more or less simultaneously, and it may be quite difficult to disentangle the effects of each one of them. Some may pull in the same direction, and may add, multiply, or interact in the production of effects. Others may counteract each other, so that an increase in X, which normally produces an increase in Y, is instead accompanied by a decrease in Y, because Z more than compensated the effects of the increase in X. For instance, increasing buying power in Norway during the last third of the nineteenth century should have produced an increase in alcohol consumption, since alcohol is (and was) income elastic. Nevertheless consumption decreased because of ideological changes (the expansion of the temperance movement), severe reductions in availability of alcohol, and the increasing availability of an alternative beverage (coffee).

This kind of situation, where a large number of variables change simultaneously, and interact in complex ways, is a normal state of affairs for substance abuse researchers at all levels. It is not limited to historians and social scientists. The clinical researcher also faces a multitude of causal factors that interact to determine — or at least influence — his clients drinking career. And the biologist faces equally complex systems, where changes in one parameter trigger series of events of different types.

In very complex causal systems, where each variable influences and is influenced by several other variables, simple questions may have very complicated answers. Changes in one variable at one instant may produce changes in several others, which interact to induce new changes in the first variable etc. Such systems are not easily studied by experimental methods, while retaining a minimum level of external validity. In order to fully grasp the essence of such processes one needs good theoretical representations of the system, for instance in the form of mathematical or other types of models. Hence, one must leave the domain of direct observation (possibly after an experimental manipulation) of each separate causal link, and study systems of such links by hypothetical-deductive methods. One may not be able to test directly each single causal link by itself, for instance because it is impossible to change only one parameter at a time. However, this is not an unusual state of affairs in science. On the contrary, in most scientific disciplines, like astronomy, geology, evolutionary biology etc. experimental manipulations are seldom possible.

In such cases, where experimental methods are not available, we have to rely on the Humean criterions of plausibility and coherence. The degree of confidence that can be obtained from plausibility and coherence, obviously depends on how well developed our theories are. The strength of theories is precisely that they can provide the frame needed to form judgements about plausibility and coherence. Theories bind together phenomena that at first sight may seem unrelated, they provide us with the mechanism needed to understand why certain relations occur and they help us to exclude many possibilities as unlikely. Therefore, the less open a field is to experimental procedures, the more strongly we need good theories.

So far, substance abuse research has not produced very advanced and general theories. Since the range of questions that experimental methods can answer is fairly limited, due to problems with the external validity of such methods, our discipline clearly needs better theories in order to develop further.

DOES EVERYTHING HAVE A CAUSE?

Determinism is the idea that everything has a cause. It can also be formulated as follows: if two closed systems are identical up to a given point in time, then they will be identical at all later times.

Twentieth century science has produced results that seriously challenge determinism. Quantum mechanics and chaos theory are well-known examples. In my view, there are also purely epistemological reasons for questioning determinism. The reasons for this are intimately tied in with the action-theoretical postulate of experimental methodology, mentioned earlier. However, I shall not go into the details of this complicated issue here.

The search for causal relationships is an integral part of science. However, when determinism is rejected as a metaphysical principle, one has to face the possibility that sometimes our search for causal explanations may be in vain. Some phenomena simply cannot be explained causally. We shall consider this possibility at two different levels — the level of individual organisms, and the aggregate level of whole societies, starting with the former.

One can choose between two different paradigms in relation to the individual organism, and in particular in relation to human behaviour. Either one can simply deny determinism, and proceed on the assumption that human behaviour cannot be completely understood within a deterministic framework. Or one may want to find an explicit argument for indeterminism at this level. Thus, if one believes that human behaviour is not completely determined, one may wish to identify where this indeterminism comes from.

If the latter strategy is chosen, one is tempted to venture the possibility that indeterminism at the level of individual organisms may be rooted in quantum mechanical indeterminacy. However, this is not at all obvious, since uncertainty at the atomic level may have no practical consequences at the macro-level. Large ensembles of particles typically tend to be deterministic at the aggregate level, although the state of each element is indeterminate.

However, there are a few possible exceptional cases, where micro-level uncertainty may tunnel through to the macro-level. Elster (1979) mentions two possible examples of such 'tunnelling'. Mutations are the 'fuel' of biological evolution, and since natural selection, or survival of the fittest,

54   The Nature of Alcohol and Drug Related Problems

takes care of the 'good' mutations, micro-level phenomena have effects at the macro-level. Perhaps some mutations may be the result of quantum mechanical or thermodynamical mechanisms. If this is true, micro-level indeterminacy produces indeterminacy at the macro-level as well. Another possible example is the neurological mechanisms underlying mental processes. Perhaps ideas — new ideas — may sometimes be triggered by quantum mechanical mechanisms in our brains. If so, one cannot expect that our behaviour can be fully accounted for by causal mechanisms.

A third candidate of 'tunnelling' can be imagined in the setting of non-linear systems in the chaotic region. Since even the smallest uncertainty gives rise to qualitatively different outcomes in such cases, objective chance at the micro-level may have large effects at the macro-level. The 'butterfly effect' is the modern term for this phenomenon. If human behaviour is regulated by non-linear (in the mathematical sense) processes in our bodies and/or non-linear interactions with the environment, then one can easily imagine that the outcome may sometimes be impossible to predict.

These mechanisms suggest that human behaviour may be predictable on the basis of causal mechanisms only within fairly narrow limits. In particular, individual drinking careers, including alcoholic drinking careers, may be quite difficult to explain and predict. This unpredictability is not necessarily a sign of our ignorance and the crudeness of our theories — it may also be a sign of an inherent indeterminacy in reality itself. Perhaps many drinking careers are chaotic processes (in the technical meaning of the word), highly sensitive to small changes in key parameters.

I shall now turn to the level of social aggregates, and ask if it can be safely presumed that all changes in aggregate level variables, such as the per capita alcohol consumption level, the prevalence of abstention, the rate of inflation, the suicide rate etc. can be explained causally. If the answer to this question is negative, it implies that cultural change cannot be predicted with confidence. Furthermore, the potentials of rational policies become severely circumscribed, since political measures can have only fairly limited effects in such a world.

It will be argued that indeterminacy at the level of individuals may produce indeterminacy even at the aggregate level, and hence that macro-level changes in some variables cannot be fully understood in terms of other macro-level variables.

A variant of this problem is the well-known question of the role of the individual in history. May the course of history be deflected by the action of a single individual? As Elster (1983) suggests, this is basically a question of societies' developmental stability or homeorhesis. They have this property if, for any small perturbation in societies' course of development they will later on resume the development they would have taken had the perturbation not occurred. If societies are stable in this sense, and if any action by an

Epistemological problems in substance abuse research 55

individual counts as a small contribution, then one could say that the individual has no proper role in history: what goes on at the micro-level, has no effect at the macro-level.

There are several reasons to question whether this can be generally true for social systems. Social systems are complex, in the sense that many different aspects interact. In general, non-linearity must be the rule and chaos theory then suggests that homeorhesis cannot always be expected under such circumstances. Small perturbations may have very large effects.

We will look at a special case of this problem somewhat more closely, and two ways of looking at it will be described. I let Durkheim represent the deterministic view. He argues that the individual has no effect on the aggregate. I shall outline a counter-argument that implies the opposite conclusion, and that allows an indeterministic view of society.

Consider an aggregate social variable — for instance the mean alcohol consumption level in society, the suicide rate etc. Such aggregate variables are arithmetical means of individual values. (In the case of the suicide rate, the individual value are equal to one if the person has committed suicide and zero in the opposite case.) In relation to such averages, Durkheim (1964, p. 8) has argued: 'Since each of these figures contains all the individual cases indiscriminately, the individual circumstances which may have had a share in the production of the phenomenon are neutralized and, consequently, do not contribute to its determination. The average, then, expresses a certain state of the group mind (l'ame collective).'

In Durkheim's perspective, the culture exists above and beyond the individuals, and exerts 'external coercive power' over them. Individual level phenomena cannot explain aggregate level averages — that is, differences between social groups and social categories, or changes over time. In short, Durkheim claims that social facts should be explained in terms of other social facts. I shall now outline this argument somewhat more closely, and will then argue against it.

Durkheim's argument, as quoted above, is based on the law of large numbers. Individual changes, say in consumption behaviour, very often occur because one gets a new job, or some new friends, because of changes in the family, because one decides to change lifestyle and re-allocate resources, or due to diseases and so forth. However, the law of large numbers should guarantee that these individual fluctuations would cancel each other out and therefore have no significant effect in the form of variations at the aggregate level, say in per capita consumption. Only when the individual changes are harmonized by an external force, would one expect changes in per capita consumption. However, in that case we are no longer talking about 'individual' fluctuations. Therefore — to paraphrase Durkheims argument — unless the law of large numbers is abolished, the 'sociological dogma' that macro-level changes should have macro-level (i.e. common) causes, ought to be valid.

Now, the important point is that the law of large numbers may not be valid for social systems. The law of large numbers basically applies to situations where the individuals act independently of each other, but this is obviously not true in social systems, since individuals influence each other's behaviour both directly and indirectly, and in many different ways.

At the level of primary social groups, where everybody influences everybody else, the law of large numbers is clearly not valid. In this case, individual-level fluctuations, that are synchronized via social interaction, would be observable at the aggregate level, i.e. in the group average.

In society at large, it is clear that everybody does not influence everybody — at least not directly. However, a society can be conceived of as an enormous social network — that is, a system of actors tied together by different types of social relations which tend to co-ordinate their behaviour. Each actor is influenced by a fairly small number of co-actors, but he is indirectly tied to a very large number of others (possibly all members of society) by mutual friends, friends of friends and so forth. In effect, one can argue that each actor is influenced by practically every other member of his culture. From the study of mathematical models of such interactive systems, it is known that these indirect connections may in fact be fairly strong, provided that the interpersonal ties exceed a certain minimum value and that the network has certain structural characteristics (Skog 1986). This has been called 'the principle of long-range indirect ties'. It implies that the law of large numbers breaks down even in very large populations.

When the principle of long-range indirect ties is valid, we would observe changes in the population average that would have no counterpart in other aggregate level variables, and hence no simple cause. Since individual fluctuations have multiple causes (which essentially must be of a social nature, having their roots in interaction), the same must be true for the corresponding fluctuations in the population average. Therefore, these changes will typically have an enormous number of micro-level causes.

If practically everyone influences, and is influenced by most members of society via indirect ties, then one should also expect the behaviour in question to be a collective behaviour. Not in the sense that everyone does the same things, but in the sense that the whole population should slide up and down the consumption scale, more or less in concert, when the population average changes. Formally, this is easily verified to be the case (Skog 1986). Hence, the same mechanisms both produce collective behaviour and allow micro-level, or individual, fluctuations to be a significant macro-level phenomenon. In this perspective the distinction between collective and individual thus appear to be more problematic than is normally presumed.

The perspective outlined above creates a picture of the culture which is well described by the metaphor of a 'boiling pot'. We 'see' an enormously complex system of actors whose behaviour is constantly modified by the behaviour of 'neighbours' in the topological space of the social network. Sociometrically local changes may remain local, or they may tend to travel through the network with the semblance of spreading waves, which mix, fortify and counteract each other. Sometimes they create aggregate changes in one direction, sometimes in the other, and sometimes they neutralize each other.

Let us take the drinking culture as an example. The argument outlined above suggests that the historical transformation of the drinking culture must, at least to some extent, be understood as a dynamic process within the drinking culture itself, and that this perspective is at least as important as an analysis in terms of independently measurable 'factors' and 'variables' with a known history. When consumption of alcoholic beverages goes up, for example because people start to drink wine, rather than water with meals, or because people begin to take beer as a thirst quencher on ordinary week days, these changes should be understood in terms of the actions and interactions of the people who actually do the drinking, and not only in terms of external influences. What actually happens, is that real human beings start to drink alcoholic beverages in situations which used to be the 'domain' of other beverages, and this habit spreads by way of social interaction between people. Sometimes such transformations may be triggered by exogenous changes, such as increased availability of alcohol or increased buying power, but this need not be the case. New habits can be born, and old habits can die out for no apparent reason, as is well known from other sectors of social life (e.g. fashions). The fact that we can see no apparent reasons is not necessarily a sign of ignorance and failure to identify the true causes. The arguments outlined above suggest that external causes may not always exist.

In conclusion, we must be open to the possibility that many phenomena may not lend themselves to causal explanations, or that we may find only partial explanations of many phenomena. Objective randomness may not be limited to the micro-cosmos of quantum mechanics — it may very well prevail at all levels.

CONCLUSION

The main points that the author has tried to substantiate on the preceding pages can be summarized as follows:

- An event is a cause of another event if the former produces or brings about the latter.

- Causation cannot be reduced to constant conjunction, or to necessary and/or sufficient conditions. In order to be able to separate causation and spurious correlation one must adopt an action-theoretical perspective. Controlled experiments allow us to distinguish between the two.
- In actual practice, however, controlled experiments can answer only a limited class of questions. Many phenomena cannot be realistically controlled or manipulated.
- With non-experimental methods it becomes difficult to separate causation and spurious correlation. By attacking the same question from different angles, and with different types of data, one can increase the likelihood of disclosing spurious correlations. Good theories and hypothetical-deductive methods also contribute to this.
- Although the search for causal explanations is a major aim in science, one must be open to the possibility that not everything can be explained causally. If indeterminism (objective chance) is acknowledged at some level (e.g. the quantum mechanical) it may also be present at higher levels, including the level of human behaviour and the level of cultural development.

REFERENCES

Anscombe, E. (1975). Causality and determination. In Sorsa, E. (ed.) *Causation and conditionals*, pp. 63–81. Oxford University Press, Oxford.
Beauchamp, T. L. and Rosenberg, A. (1981). *Hume and the problem of causation*. Oxford University Press, Oxford.
Box, G. E. P. and Jenkins, G. M. (1976). *Time series analysis: forecasting and control* (revised Edn). Holden-Day, San Francisco.
Durkheim, E. (1964). *The rules of sociological method*. Free Press, New York.
Elster, J. (1979). *Forklaring og dialektikk*, Pax, Oslo.
Elster, J. (1983). *Explaining technical change*. Cambridge University Press, London.
Glymour, C. (1986). Statistics and metaphysics. *Journal of the American Statistical Association*, **81**, 964–6.
Holland, P. (1986). Statistics and causal inference. *Journal of the American Statistical Association*, **81**, 945–60.
Lewis, D. (1973). Causation. *Journal of Philosophy*, **70**, 556–67.
Lieberson, S. (1985). *Making it count*. University of California Press, Berkeley.
Palmer, T. (1989). A weather eye on unpredictability. *New Scientist*, **11**, Nov. 56–9.
Pedersen, W. (1990). Foreldre som 'alkohollangere'? *Tidsskrift for den Norske Lægeforening*, **110**, 1834–7.
Skog, O.-J. (1986). The long waves of alcohol consumption: a social network perspective on cultural change. *Social Networks*, **8**, 1–32.
Skog, O.-J. (1988). Testing causal hypotheses about correlated trends: pitfalls and remedies. *Contemporary Drug Problems*, **15**, 565–606.

Suppes, P. (1970). *A probabilistic theory of causation*. North-Holland, Amsterdam.
Wilson, K. (1979). Problems in physics with many scales of length. *Scientific American*, **241**, 140–57, August.
Wright, G. H. von (1971). *Explanation and understanding*. Routledge and Kegan Paul, London.

4

Problems and dependence: chalk and cheese or bread and butter?

D. COLIN DRUMMOND

INTRODUCTION

The 'problems' concept, albeit under different guises, has been an essential component of theories of addiction for several centuries. That the use of psychoactive substances is associated with a wide range of severe and costly problems has long provided a rationale for societal concern and more recently for expenditure on treatment services for substance misusers. Harmless substance use would deserve considerably less attention.

In his *Enquiry into the Effects of Spiritous Liquors on the Human Body*, Rush (1785) linked the consumption of certain alcoholic drinks to the gradual emergence of increasingly severe physical, psychiatric, and social adverse consequences. Moral and physical deterioration were, in his view, caused by the type rather than the alcohol content of the beverage (the latter now being the prevailing view) and the quantity and frequency of its use. Nevertheless, this causal explanation provided a focus for societal concern about alcohol and a rationale for the emergent Temperance Movement. Such a disaggregated view of problems relating to drinking engendered a moralistic view of inebriety. In contrast, the subsequent growth in popularity of a disease concept of alcoholism in the late nineteenth century led to a shift towards medical 'ownership' and a more compassionate view of sufferers.

Although the Temperance Movement chose such an interpretation, Rush's essay also included an early exposition of a disease theory of addiction and a description of the co-ocurrence of symptoms which are now viewed as part of the alcohol dependence syndrome (Edwards and Gross 1976). He described craving, salience of drink-seeking behaviour, loss of control over alcohol intake, and morning withdrawal symptoms: all important components of the dependence syndrome. A crucial distinction between the views of earlier theorists and Edwards and Gross, however, is in the latter's suggestion that the symptoms of dependence should be seen as

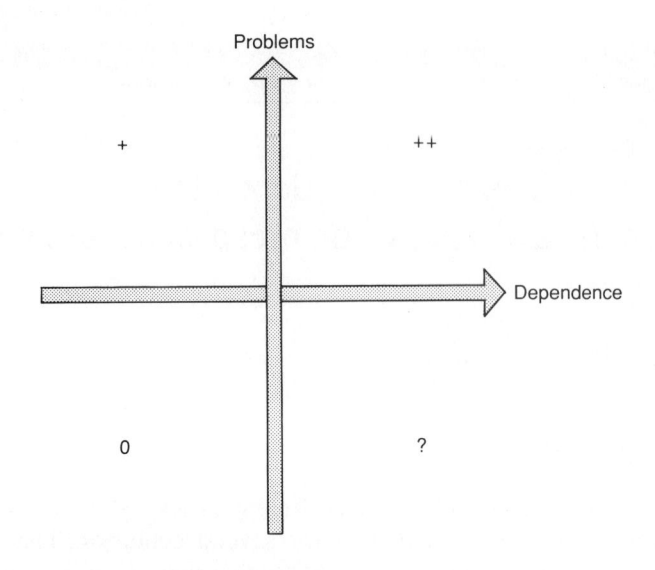

FIG. 4.1 The bi-axial concept.

conceptually separate from problems. This bi-axial concept, originally put forward by a WHO scientific group (Edwards *et al.* 1977) raises the possibility that one could experience problems in the absence of a significant degree of dependence on a substance and vice versa.

Figure 4.1 is a diagrammatic representation of this proposed relationship between the problems and dependence dimensions. Four quadrants are present between the two axes. The lower left quadrant represents a group in the population who take a substance but experience neither significant dependence nor problems. The upper right quadrant identifies a group who experience both dependence and problems, a group typically seen in a clinical setting. In the upper left quadrant are those who experience problems related to non-dependent use of the substance, an example of which would be the young, inexperienced drinker who is not significantly dependent on alcohol but is over-represented in, for example, alcohol-related road traffic accidents. Finally, the lower right quadrant represents those who are significantly dependent but do not experience problems: a 'harmless' dependence. This is unlikely to occur in the case of alcohol but the therapeutic use of nicotine chewing gum can be viewed as probably less harmful than smoking tobacco. It is important to note that these quadrants do not represent distinct categories, since as has been suggested, problems and dependence lie on continua of severity rather than representing all-or-nothing phenomena (Edwards *et al.* 1977). So the suggestion is, that problems and dependence might occur independently and in different degrees.

Other chapters in this book study the definition of the problems concept, it's associations and possible causes. This paper will explore two further important questions: (1) how might problems and dependence differ conceptually? and (2) what is the statistical relationship between problems and dependence in empirical studies?

THE PRACTICAL IMPORTANCE OF PROBLEMS AND DEPENDENCE

Before exploring these questions it is important to briefly rehearse the reason why these matters might be of concern to clinicians or researchers. First it is important that we should all agree on what it is we are talking about. To say that a study 'involved 100 alcoholics' or 'this addict requires . . .' is little better than saying 'I would like some groceries delivered' and 'my address is somewhere in the Northern Hemisphere'. Clearly, diagnostic and classification systems must aim to be specific about the nature of addiction as well as, obviously, other disorders.

Second, a move from a unitary view of addiction towards a bi-axial concept opens up the possibility of more appropriate matching of treatments to individual needs. Problem drinkers and drug takers come to treatment not only with different aspirations and motivation but with different kinds of problem. These differences require management which is sensitive to individual needs, rather than the blanket application of poorly focused approaches. An understanding of the relationship between problems and dependence could potentially introduce a greater degree of scientific precision into an imperfect art.

Thirdly, the bi-axial concept opens up a completely new research agenda. A view of alcoholics as a heterogeneous group, differing along several dimensions prompts a re-evaluation of earlier research. The importance of the dependence syndrome in clinical research has been reviewed by Edwards (1986). In the ten year period reviewed by Edwards, there have been numerous examples of the predictive value of the dependence concept. An important example is the finding that responsiveness to alcohol-related cues (Hodgson *et al.* 1979) and perception of cues for drinking (Rankin *et al.* 1982) are related to degree of dependence. Further, degree of dependence has been found to have important implications for the long term outcome of alcoholism (Edwards *et al.* 1983). These and other studies provide compelling evidence not only for changes in the psychobiological state associated with different degrees of dependence but also underline the potential importance of dependence in studies of treatment and relapse.

In contrast, the problems dimension has received relatively less attention, possibly in part due to the difficulties associated with its measurement.

A recent treatment study found, however, that alcohol-related problems were the only factor which suggested the superiority of 'extended treatment' over 'advice' at two year follow-up (Chick et al. 1988).

PROBLEMS AND DEPENDENCE: SIMILARITIES AND DIFFERENCES

Problems and dependence are similar in the sense that they are both disabilities associated with the consumption of a substance. Dependence can be viewed as a special kind of problem involving an altered psychobiological state and is by definition, intrapersonal. Most problems however, are interpersonal: they can best be seen as arising from an interaction between the individual's behaviour associated with drug use and societal reactions towards it (Jessor and Jessor 1977). Clearly there are notable exceptions to this general principle, largely occurring in the realm of physical pathology (e.g. hepatic cirrhosis, cerebral damage, accidents etc.) and mental illness (e.g. depression and anxiety). Nevertheless, most problems are common human experiences which may often arise in the absence of drug or alcohol use, and thus are perhaps more easily perceived and understood. Dependence on the other hand represents a rather special relationship between a drug and a drug taker. In this sense, we 'know' what problems are, but we do not 'know' what dependence is.

Time course

(a) Event vs process

A further important conceptual distinction between problems and dependence lies in the time course of the two phenomena. Certain problems are best seen as 'events' occurring from time to time in an individual's drug taking career. Take, for example, the problem of a conviction for drunk driving. The convicted person may have driven a car whilst under the influence of alcohol on many occasions without any adverse consequences. On the particular evening of his arrest, however, a co-occurrence of particular circumstances (an accident, the arrival of the police, detection of an excess serum alcohol level and a successful conviction) gave rise to the 'problem'. At each point in the chain of events an unremarkable evening became increasingly problematic (although, clearly, the point at which the drinker got into the car marked the onset of a potential problem for himself and others). Such a problem may coexist with other problems such as a marital or financial problem. This clustering of problems does not necessarily reflect connections between problems as part of an evolving process, although the problem events may share a common cause, excessive alcohol consumption.

Dependence on the other hand is best seen as an evolving process. Unlike the problem of a drunk driving conviction, dependence does not arise suddenly one evening. From the point at which an individual takes the first dose of a drug the process of physiological and psychological adaptation to the drug begins. The process of neuroadaptation and the reinforcing effects of drugs together lead to gradual emergence of dependence. The development of withdrawal symptoms provides motivation for relief drug taking leading to increased tolerance. Thus dependence symptoms are intimately linked.

(b) Transience

Another distinction between problems and dependence in relation to the time dimension concerns the relative transience of problems. Cahalan's (1970) general population follow-up survey suggested that having alcohol-related problems at one time, is a poor predictor of problems at a later date. This may be related to the combination of the narrow time frame of survey methods and the infrequency of occurrence of certain problems. For example, Macdonald and Pederson (1988) found that in a clinical population of problem drinkers, the probability of being arrested for drunk driving was approximately once every 1168 impaired driving events, or once every 9–10 years. The apparent disappearance of problems over time found in surveys may even reflect a lack of validity in the methods used to measure problems.

Room (1977) has suggested that drinking problems seen in the general population may occupy a different 'world' from the more established and chronic problems observed in clinical populations. This has led to a dichotomy between clinicians' and survey researchers' views of problems.

The transience of alcohol-related problems may also indicate a further difference between problems and dependence. Although this has not been systematically studied it appears that dependence tends to increase progressively over time. While dependence can progress and regress throughout a lifetime it seems probable that beyond a certain degree of dependence this variability declines, until in the severely dependent, a return to drug use after a period of abstinence results in reinstatement to a pre-abstinent pattern of consumption and dependence symptoms (Edwards and Gross 1976). As dependence becomes more established, the relationship between the individual and the drug in most cases becomes permanently altered. Follow-up of alcoholics in the long term lends support to this view (Edwards *et al.* 1983), with few severely dependent drinkers able to return to a lasting social drinking pattern.

Problems do not occur in such an orderly manner. Objectively severe problems may occur many years before less severe ones. A severe problem may occur early in a drug taking career and never arise again throughout the individual's lifetime.

Causality

So far, this analysis has assumed a causal relationship between the consumption of a drug and the development of a problem. In practice, however, it is often extremely difficult to establish such a causal connection (Room 1977). Clearly this can be affected by a number of factors, notably the attributions of the survey respondent. This difficulty led Edwards *et al.* (1977) pessimistically to suggest that 'The assumptions on which such a determination might be based would usually be so dubious that, wherever possible, a search for causes should be avoided.' (p. 7) In practice, questionnaires and interviews employed in surveys have tended to rely on the subject's view of the alcohol-relatedness of their problems (Edwards *et al.* 1973; Cahalan and Room 1974; Makela and Simpura 1985; Hilton 1987*a*). Nevertheless, the question of causality may hold the key to some important conceptual similarities as well as differences between problems and dependence.

Consider the following situation. A man who is in an unhappy marriage begins to spend an increasing amount of time in a bar on his way home from work. His conscious or unconscious motivation may be to avoid the spouse in whose company he feels unhappy. He may find solace in the company of others who share similar sentiments. In order to pass the time and to avoid feeling left out he may drink an increasing amount of alcohol before returning home. On his return home, disinhibited by alcohol, he becomes increasingly short-tempered with his wife and arguments ensue over his expenditure of their joint funds on alcohol. As a result, the following night he fails to come home until the bar closes and his drinking escalates. This is an example of a positive feedback loop: the more he drinks, the more his home life becomes unpleasant leading to more drinking (Fig. 4.2).

At the same time a similar process may be occurring in relation to his dependence on alcohol. His alcohol consumption affords at least temporary relief from unpleasant mood states. As tolerance develops, so more alcohol is required to bring about relief. As withdrawal symptoms begin to emerge, his drinking begins to be directed towards their relief until he starts to drink in the morning to avoid the onset of withdrawal symptoms: another positive feedback loop. Both processes can, independently, explain the reinforcing effect of alcohol for this unfortunate man.

At the point of seeking help in an Alcohol Treatment Unit, his stated

```
Marital problem ─────→ Alcohol consumption ─────→ Intoxication
      ↑                          |
      └──────────────────────────┘


Alcohol consumption ─────→ ↑ Tolerance
      ↑                          |
      └──────────────────────────┘
```

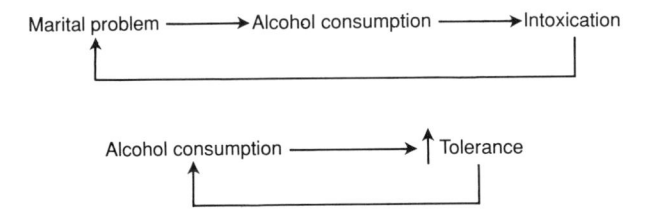

FIG. 4.2 Causal mechanisms in the development of problems and dependence.

reason for doing so was his marital problem, blaming his wife for her lack of empathy. His wife, however, keen to set the record straight pointed out that his previous marriage had foundered due to his drinking and aggressiveness, and that early in the current relationship he was often drunk even when the situation called for restraint. An early example included their wedding.

As the history further unfolded, his mother was able to confirm that his father and paternal grandfather had both experienced severe drinking problems.

His story is the 'bread and butter' of everyday clinical work and yet it illustrates the complexities in attempting to unravel causes of problems and dependence. Numerous alternative interpretations can be made of the interaction between the influences which have helped to bring him to this point in his drinking career. Much will depend on the attributions of the observer. His strong family history could be viewed as providing a genetic predisposition to develop dependence or alternatively, on a psychodynamic level, as a predisposing factor in his current acting-out of the conflicts with his forebears. In the latter case his choice of unsuitable partners is a symptom of his conflict, whereas in the former, an unfavourable marriage could be seen as an important factor mediating the development of dependence.

Clearly problems and dependence arise out of a complex interplay between the individual, the drug, and the environment, which is not easily understood in our current state of knowledge. One can begin, however, by proposing different mechanisms for their development. Even within the problems domain their may be different mechanisms responsible for the development of different problems. Relatively mild and infrequent exposure to alcohol at lunchtime could result in problems at work in occupations which involve the operation of dangerous machinery, whereas occasional heavy weekend drinking in young males may lead to an excess of road traffic accidents, and injuries due to fights, in association with low tolerance to alcohol. Severe dependence on the other hand may require more prolonged high levels of exposure to alcohol for its development, a causal pathway which it may share with certain physical pathologies such as hepatic cirrhosis. While such causal hypotheses make intuitive sense they cannot be assumed to be correct. But, as the author will endeavour to show later, statistical methods can usefully be employed in exploring causal models of problems and dependence.

Vulnerability

Research into life events (Brown and Harris 1978) and alcohol-related problems have much in common in that they are both concerned with adverse experiences in relation to mental disorders. They differ, however, in the proposed direction of causality: life events causing mental illness or drinking behaviour in the former and drinking behaviour causing problems in the latter. Similar difficulties in establishing the direction of causality (as described above) have been experienced in determining the independence of life events. It is therefore unsurprising that the extension of a life events methodology into the addiction field has proved extremely difficult (Cooke and Allan 1984).

The concept of vulnerability has been used to describe the factors which mediate the effects of life events, on the expression of mental disorder in the individual. Similarly, the expression of drug- or alcohol-related problems could be mediated by vulnerability factors such as socio-economic status, social supports, age, sex, personality, nutrition, or physical and mental health (Jellinek 1960; Langenbucher and Nathan 1983; Sadava 1985). Further it is possible that the expression of problems and dependence (or indeed different kinds of problem) may be mediated by different vulnerability factors.

The pathoplastic influence of culture

Cultural differences in the development of problems and dependence interested Jellinek (1960). He described five species of alcoholism: alpha, beta, gamma, delta, and epsilon. He suggested that, based on cultural stereotypes, Anglo-Saxon drinkers would tend towards gamma alcoholism, experiencing both problems and dependence, whereas continental drinkers would tend to experience dependence with few problems (delta). These species, although representing all-or-nothing phenomena, bear a similarity to the concepts displayed in Fig. 4.1. Figure 4.3 shows Jellinek's species superimposed on the problems and dependence axes (the solid arrows between species indicate transitions proposed by Jellinek. The broken arrow indicates a possible, although infrequent, transition).

Beta alcoholism he viewed as the experience of certain problems without dependence due to cultural susceptibility to the effects of alcohol. Alpha

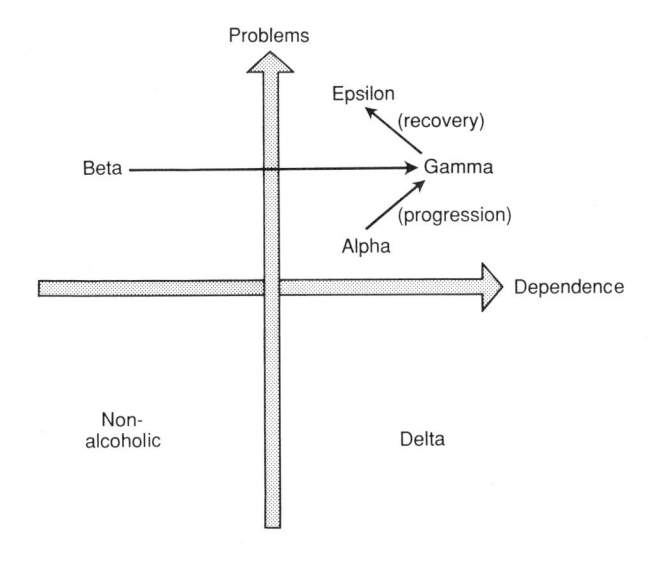

FIG. 4.3 Jellinek's typologies of alcoholism.

alcoholics, he referred to as being typical 'problem drinkers', although the co-occurrence of 'psychological' dependence and some problems, allies this group more to gamma than delta. In fact he viewed alpha as being in some cases a precursor of gamma. From Jellinek's brief description, it is not clear exactly where in this scheme, epsilon alcoholics fall. It is implied that they represent a group of partially recovered gamma alcoholics who, during drinking bouts, experience serious problems but whose dependence is not as marked as in gamma alcoholism. This would ally epsilon more to beta than gamma. To further complicate matters, however, he viewed epsilon as a form of relapse into gamma alcoholism.

While his formulation was based on stereotypes rather than empirical findings this analysis underlines the importance of cross-cultural comparisons of the relationship between problems and dependence.

Edwards *et al.* (1977) expanded the analysis of the effect of cultural influences on the development of problems. They suggested that problems must be viewed in the social and cultural context in which they occur, since many problems arise through a discrepancy between the individual's drinking behaviour and the prevailing societal norms. Behaviour which is at odds with such norms attracts social disapproval, bringing the individual into conflict with society. In Muslim cultures any drinking attracts severe penalties, whereas in certain parts of Western Europe even regular morning drinking is quite acceptable, if not, actively encouraged.

The drug and its mode of presentation

As suggested earlier, Rush (1785) attributed different problems to different modes of presentation of alcohol. With the benefit of hindsight, his attribution would now be seen as incorrect although his observation was accurate. Possibly the more severely dependent eighteenth century drinker sought out the more potent preparation as is the case in his late twentieth century counterpart. Rush's suggestion, however has much to be commended. The mode of presentation of a drug often determines the problems which ensue. Dependence may also be influenced by the mode of presentation, although perhaps to a lesser extent. Methods of administration which bring about a more rapid onset of drug effects, tend to lead to a more rapid development of dependence.

In relation to drug comparisons, problems tend to be generally rather drug specific whereas commonalities are more easily found in the expression of dependence. Dependence on barbiturates and alcohol, for example, is remarkably similar, whereas the physical complications caused by these two classes of drug are very different.

ARE PROBLEMS AND DEPENDENCE THEORETICALLY RELATED?

So far we have focused on the possible differences between problems and dependence phenomena. There are clearly several reasons to suppose that they might occur independently in different degrees, as suggested by the bi-axial concept. They also, as has been suggested, share a common cause: alcohol consumption. Heavier consumption should lead to more problems and a higher degree of dependence. But could dependence influence problems or vice versa?

To explore this question, let us return to the example of our luckless drinker. Whatever the initial causes of his heavy drinking, he now has an established and high degree of dependence. He experiences withdrawal symptoms throughout the day, for which he takes regular doses of alcohol from a bottle which he carries to work in his brief-case. His repertoire of drinking, in other words, has become extremely narrow. He drinks every day irrespective of the time of day or the social situation in which he finds himself; at work, at home, while driving a car, as well as in the pub. This hazardous drinking pattern brings him into contact with considerable social disapproval (e.g. losing his job, his wife leaving him, and a drunk driving conviction). His friend, with whom he sometimes drinks at weekends, consumes exactly the same amount of alcohol in a month, but has a very different drinking pattern. He drinks heavily at weekends, staying at friends houses when drunk, and when he is on holiday. His repertoire of drinking remains sufficiently flexible that he is able to plan his drinking in such a way that he will avoid much of the social disapproval to which his friend is susceptible (he does not drink at or before work, he always takes public transport on drinking days, and makes sure that he does not return home drunk to his wife). He is therefore able to experience fewer problems.

Clearly, the friend is not problem-free. His dependence is likely to escalate, therefore increasing the probability of experiencing the consequent social opprobrium. His current pattern of drinking may, even at this point, place him at a higher risk than his friend for other types of problem such as injuries or asphyxiation due to inhalation of vomit whilst intoxicated. Nevertheless, there is the theoretical possibility that the two drinkers may experience different levels of problems consequent upon their different degrees of dependence. In addition, the severely dependent drinker may have experienced fewer problems at an earlier stage in his drinking career, not necessarily because he drank less, but possibly also because he was less dependent. Thus he was previously able to schedule his drinking in a more socially acceptable way.

The possibility that dependence might in some way be important in mediating the development of problems has been succinctly stated by Edwards *et al.* (1977).

The individual's drinking may arouse suspicion because it is no longer in accord with cultural expectations, in terms not only of quantity drunk but of the timing and occasions of drinking.... The daily pattern [of drinking] he establishes is typically one which ensures the maintenance of a relatively high blood alcohol throughout the waking period and the avoidance of withdrawal. In a culture where drinking is easily accepted, this goal may be achieved without offending any cultural proscriptions, but where the basic cultural pattern is of more spaced drinking (typically perhaps only at the end of the day), the individual who is scheduling his drinking so as to maintain his desired blood alcohol level may face a difficult daily logistic problem, may easily offend against cultural norms, and may have to drink according to a less set and predictable pattern.

Could a causal relationship in the opposite direction be postulated, i.e. could problems theoretically cause dependence? It is possible that problems provide a positive feedback loop to consumption and hence, dependence, (as suggested above) but it is intuitively much less likely that problems should directly influence dependence. One example might include the onset of the problem of brain injury through heavy alcohol consumption leading to loss of tolerance, but this is clearly in the opposite direction of effect.

ARE PROBLEMS AND DEPENDENCE STATISTICALLY RELATED?

While conceptual differences exist between problems and dependence, is the bi-axial concept supported by empirical evidence? It seems intuitively likely that increasing levels of alcohol consumption should be associated with a greater number and severity of problems. This view is certainly born out by general population studies which have examined the relationship between per capita alcohol consumption and, for example, mortality from hepatic cirrhosis. It is equally possible, however, that other factors described above, including dependence, may mediate the consumption-problems relationship.

Basic considerations

Before examining empirical evidence, however, it is essential to bear in mind that the presence or absence of a statistical correlation between empirically measured phenomena does not necessarily imply a causal relationship (a point which has been clearly made by both Kreitman and Skog in this volume, see p. 99 and p. 37). Indeed, the conceptual differences described above are alone, sufficient to justify the existence of the bi-axial concept (Drummond 1990). It is important, therefore, to examine what a correlation might tell us about causal relationships. Kenny (1979) suggests that in empirical research 'causal modelling can assist in the development, modification, and extension of measurement and substantive theory'. Without statistical analysis, causal models remain purely theoretical speculation. Nevertheless, Kenny goes on to identify three basic conditions, relating to what is already known about the relationship between variables, which must be fulfilled before a causal relationship can be inferred.

1. Time precedence
2. Relationship
3. Non-spuriousness

1. Time precedence

Before we can infer that a correlation between alcohol consumption and problems indicates that the former causes the latter, it has to be demonstrated that the consumption occurred before the problem developed. This seems an inherently reasonable assumption to make, but in survey research these two variables are usually measured cross-sectionally. A stronger design would be to examine the onset of a problem in previously non-problematic drinkers or to introduce an experimental manipulation. It would be premature, however, to write-off cross-sectional survey methods on the basis that they are imperfect in at least one respect. Such research remains important in theory refinement. In the data which follows, the assumption is made that consumption temporally preceded problems and dependence, and that what is being observed is a state of equilibrium in a cross-sectional survey.

2. Relationship

The examination of a statistical correlation between two variables is an accepted method used to determine the existence of a relationship. This is conventionally supplemented by an estimate of statistical probability to assess the extent to which such a correlation could have occurred by chance. This does not address the issue of validity of the measures, nor is it a substitute for experimentation (although, here too there are difficulties) but does provide a standard, and widely-employed method used in much of social science and medical research to test theoretical models.

3. Non-spuriousness

The third condition described by Kenny relates to Suppes (1970) probabilistic theory of causation, which has also been discussed by Skog (Chapter 3, p. 48). If a correlation between two variables disappears when a third variable is controlled, the correlation is said to be spurious. It may also be an indication that the third variable is an intervening variable. Path analysis provides a sophisticated and widely used method for exploring the spuriousness of correlations between variables, or the existence of an intervening variable. This type of analysis assumes particular importance in studying the relationships between problems, dependence and consumption, as will be shown below, where there are theoretical grounds to suspect that dependence may represent an intervening variable in the consumption-problems relationship.

In summary, while the existence of a correlation does not necessarily indicate a causal relationship, multiple regression and path analysis provide the social scientist with useful tools to explore theory. Just as there is danger in drawing unwarranted conclusions from such analyses, so too, there is a danger in prematurely rejecting correlational analysis. Multiple regression analysis remains an essential first step in theory development and refinement.

Previous research

Several studies in clinical populations support the view that alcoholism is statistically multidimensional (Polich et al. 1981; Skinner 1981; Wanberg and Horn 1983; Hesselbrock et al. 1983). Babor et al. (1988) have recently reviewed the evidence concerning the dimensionality of alcoholism in terms of problems and dependence by looking at treatment outcome studies. They concluded that the evidence does not clearly support either a unitary or a multidimensional view. A similar division of opinion exists over the relationship between problems and dependence in the case of other drugs, with some supporting (Sadava 1985; Kosten et al. 1987; Skinner and Goldberg 1986) and others arguing against (Hasin et al. 1988) a multidimensional view. Further, there is some support for the view that alcohol consumption may represent a third, independent dimension (Sadava 1985; Skinner 1988).

It was against this background that a study which will be described was conducted in three London hospitals (the Maudsley, Priory, and Stone House Hospitals) (Drummond 1990). The Severity of Alcohol Dependence Questionnaire (SADQ) (Stockwell et al. 1979) provides a useful and reliable means of measuring alcohol dependence, but it's relationship to the problems dimension was unknown. This questionnaire consists of 20 items relating to the alcohol dependence syndrome (Edwards and Gross 1976), 4 of which relate to alcohol consumption. These latter items are considered separately as a quantity/frequency measure of alcohol consumption for the purpose of this study.

Because of the absence of a suitable instrument covering a comprehensive range of problem domains and at the same time excluding dependence items, a new instrument was devised: the Alcohol Problems Questionnaire (APQ). The items were mainly derived from the Troubles with Drinking Questionnaire (Edwards et al. 1972) and pilot interviews with patients and clinicians. Some items are similar to the Alcohol Use Inventory (Wanberg and Horn 1983). The APQ consists of 46 items (2 items have subsequently been dropped because of infrequency of reporting) covering a wide range of problem domains: friends (4), physical (7), psychological (5), police (3), finances (4), marital (9), children (6), and work (8). The two items which were dropped came from the children subscale. A total of 23 items covering the first 5 subscales are applicable to all subjects giving a 'common' subscale, the aggregate of which provides the APQ common (APQC) score. The results reported here refer only to this latter subscale.

The questionnaires were administered to 104 problem drinkers at first contact in the outpatient clinic, or as soon as possible thereafter if they were intoxicated or experiencing withdrawal symptoms. None of the subjects approached refused to participate, but one subject completed the questionnaires incorrectly, leaving a sample of 103. Demographic and social data were also collected.

The relationship between dependence, problems, and consumption

The correlations between problems, as represented by the APQC score, the SADQ score excluding consumption items, and the consumption subscale are shown in Fig. 4.4. All three measures were highly significantly correlated with each other. However, the situation is rather different with the partial correlations (Fig. 4.5). Dependence and consumption remain highly significantly correlated when problems are controlled for ($r = 0.53, p < 0.001$). Similarly, controlling for consumption, problems and dependence are still significantly correlated ($r = 0.45, p < 0.001$). The relationship between problems and consumption, controlling for dependence, however, is insignificant ($r = 0.15$, n.s.). This suggests that the highly significant relationship between problems and dependence exists independently of the quantity of alcohol consumed and that dependence may represent an intervening variable in the consumption–problems relationship. We will return to the significance of this finding later.

Could it be the case that certain problem areas were more closely related to dependence than others? It is possible that the problems represented by this questionnaire were heterogeneous. Several methods have been used to explore this question, but the one which will be described next is a principal components analysis. Separate subscale scores were computed for each of the problem domains within the common subscale. Further, subscale scores originally described by Stockwell et al. (1979) were calculated for the SADQ. These subscales, including the consumption subscale, were entered into a principal components analysis which yielded three factors, one large and two smaller factors which together accounted for 68.7 per cent of the variance (43.8 per cent, 14.3 per cent, 10.6 per cent).

An oblique rotation gave the best separation of items. The factor loadings are shown in Table 4.1. The first factor contains all the SADQ subscales, excluding affective withdrawal symptoms. It also contains the physical and financial problems subscales. This factor we will call Physical. The second factor contains only affective withdrawal symptoms from the SADQ and psychological problems (which include depression and suicidal thoughts) and problems with friends. This factor has been labelled Affective. The third factor contains only police problems, which are clearly unrelated to either dependence or other problems. Other correlates of police problems will be referred to later.

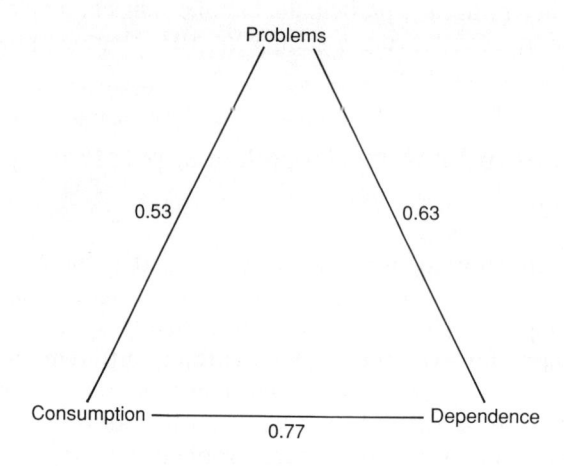

FIG. 4.4 Correlations between problems, dependence, and consumption.

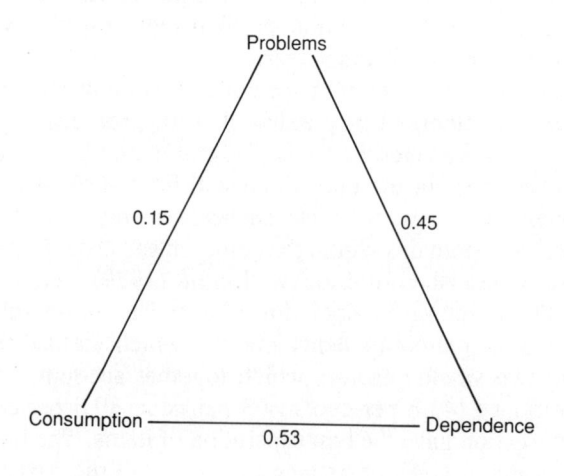

FIG. 4.5 Partial correlations between problems, dependence, and consumption.

Overall this analysis suggests that while there is a correlation between aggregate problems and dependence scores, certain problems are more closely related to particular aspects of dependence than others. Further, these statistical relationships are conceptually congruent.

TABLE 4.1 *Principal component loadings of the APQ and SADQ subscales*

	Factor 1 (Physical)	Factor 2 (Affective)	Factor 3 (Police)
APQ			
Friends	−0.17	<u>0.86</u>	0.10
Physical	<u>0.56</u>	0.14	0.32
Psychological	0.11	<u>0.74</u>	0.10
Financial	<u>0.70</u>	−0.12	0.39
Police	−0.05	0.16	<u>0.90</u>
SADQ			
Physical withdrawal	<u>0.90</u>	0.00	−0.11
Affective withdrawal	0.41	<u>0.63</u>	−0.22
Relief drinking	<u>0.86</u>	0.02	−0.12
Reinstatement	<u>0.77</u>	−0.04	−0.09
Consumption	<u>0.63</u>	0.31	−0.14

Vulnerability

General population surveys suggest that we might be likely to find differences in the number of problems experienced by different age, sex and social class groups. If so, this might indicate that social and demographic variables influence vulnerability to develop alcohol-related problems. Three separate analytic strategies were adopted to explore this question, each involving regression analysis.

First, the problems score (APQC score) was regressed on variables representing age, sex and socio-economic class. Dependence and consumption scores were included in the analysis. Dependence accounted for the greatest amount of variance in problems (Beta = 0.60, $p < 0.0001$) followed by age (Beta = −0.27, $p < 0.002$) and social class (Beta = −0.20, $p < 0.02$). Sex and the quantity of alcohol consumed did not predict problems. This suggests that younger subjects of lower socio-economic class are more likely to develop problems irrespective of their level of consumption, degree of dependence, or sex. The lack of a gender effect when consumption is controlled for has previously been noted (Mäkelä and Simpura, 1985; Hilton, 1987*b*).

Next, in order to explore whether these overall results concealed a differential effect for different problem areas, each problem subscale was regressed on the same variables. Differential effects were indeed found. Problems with friends were only predicted by the level of consumption (Beta = 0.33, $p < 0.002$) and physical problems were only predicted by dependence (Beta = 0.49, $p < 0.0001$). Psychological problems, however were predicted by dependence (Beta = 0.50, $p < 0.0001$) and sex (Beta =

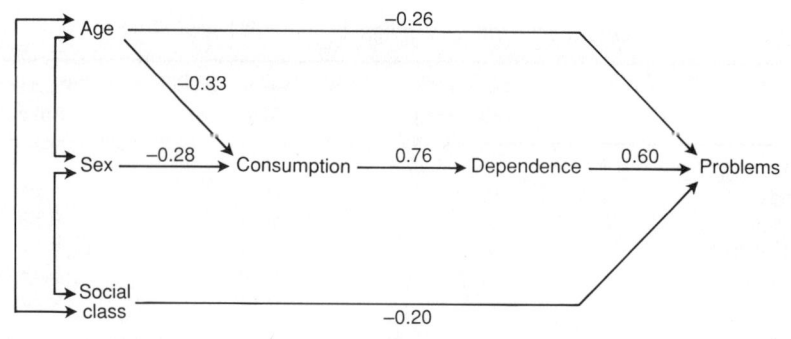

78   The Nature of Alcohol and Drug Related Problems

FIG. 4.6 Interrelationships between problems, dependence, consumption, and socio-demographic variables.

0.26, $p < 0.009$), suggesting that females are more susceptible to affective problems related to drinking. Financial problems were positively related to dependence (Beta = 0.54, $p < 0.0001$) and negatively to social class (Beta = −0.24, $p < 0.01$), indicating perhaps unsurprisingly, a susceptibility to financial problems in lower social class subjects whose drive to obtain alcohol outstrips their financial resources. Sex and social class alone predicted police problems, although these results were only marginally significant (Beta = 0.20, $p < 0.05$, Beta = −0.21, $p < 0.07$) in the direction of being male and of lower social class predicting police problems.

Finally, and most importantly, a path analysis was constructed of the interrelationships between problems, dependence, consumption, and the social and demographic variables. A series of regression analyses were performed on the variables to build a picture of the direction and strength of the relationships between the different variables (Fig. 4.6). For the sake of simplicity only the significant interrelationships between the variables have been included in the diagram.

In the centre of the diagram are problems, dependence, and consumption. Dependence, as suggested earlier predicts problems independently of consumption, and this relationship is relatively strong. As explained above, a logical assumption has been made that consumption must precede problems and that a state of equilibrium has been reached. Because of the insignificant direct relationship between consumption and problems, this places dependence as an intervening variable. Age, sex, and social class are also included in the path diagram as predictor variables since, with the possible exception of social class, it is illogical that causality could have occurred in the opposite direction i.e. consumption leading to sex or age.

The paths leading to problems are as described above. The only factor which predicts dependence is consumption, again very strongly. The sociodemographic variables have a lesser influence on problems, but are nevertheless significant. Social class is not related to consumption or to dependence, but does predict problems independently. Being male predicts a higher level of consumption, but does not directly influence problems. Lower age, however, predicts both consumption and problems independently.

CONCLUSIONS

At the start of this chapter it was suggested that problems and dependence can be seen as conceptually distinct. The data suggest that, at least in a clinical population, people who are more dependent experience more problems, but that certain problems are more closely related to particular aspects of dependence than others, which lends further empirical support to the biaxial concept. The data also support the view that people who consume more alcohol are more dependent and experience more problems. This is certainly not at odds with either previous epidemiological or clinical research, or common experience.

The new finding of interest, however, is that dependence may in some way intervene or mediate the consumption-problems relationship. This lends support to the view put forward by Edwards *et al.* (1977) that the altered behavioural state occasioned by the development of alcohol dependence may lead the drinker's pattern of alcohol consumption, in terms of both quantity drunk and the timing of drinking occasions, to become out of step with cultural expectations of 'normal' drinking behaviour. This in turn may lead to social opprobrium which forms the basis of many, if not most, alcohol-related problems. Thus, although one must be cautious about drawing unwarranted assumptions from correlational data, in this case at least there is an accord between theory and empirical findings.

Further, the data support the view that socio-demographic factors might be involved in mediating the development of problems. Different problems may be subject to different mediating factors. Dependence, on the other hand does not appear to be directly influenced by the socio-demographic factors studied here, except inasmuch as it is influenced by consumption which is independently influenced by age and sex. It is possible that other social factors mediate dependence.

It could be argued that it would be wrong to draw firm conclusions from this one small clinical study, based on a highly selected population in one European city. Research recently completed using the same instruments translated into German and administered to a German clinical population (Drummond and John, in preparation), and using similar instruments in a North American general population sample (Drummond, in preparation), point to broadly similar conclusions concerning the relationships between problems, dependence and alcohol consumption.

This work must be seen as the first step in theory testing, however. Cross-substance research on problems and dependence and the use of longitudinal and experimental research designs represent the logical next step. Further, a more fine-grained analysis is needed to explore the relationships between these variables at an individual level. The only certainty, at present, is that problems and dependence are more like bread and butter than chalk and cheese: better taken together than apart but easier to define than to separate.

REFERENCES

Babor, T. F., Dolinsky, Z., Rounsaville, B., and Jaffe, J. (1988). Unitary versus multidimensional models of alcoholism treatment outcome: an empirical study. *Journal of Studies on Alcohol*, **49**, 167–77.

Brown, G. W. and Harris, T. O. (1978). *Social origins of depression*, Tavistock, London.

Cahalan, D. (1970). *Problem drinkers: a national survey*. Jossey Bass, San Francisco.

Cahalan, D. and Cisin, I. H. (1976). Drinking behaviour and drinking problems in the United States. In Kissin, B. and Begleiter, H. (eds) *The biology of alcoholism*. Plenum, New York.

Cahalan, D. and Room, R. (1974). *Problem drinking among American men*, Rutgers Center of Alcohol Studies, Monograph No. 7. New Brunswick, New Jersey.

Chick, J., Ritson, B., Connaughton, J., Stewart, A. and Chick, J. (1988). Advice versus extended treatment for alcoholism: a controlled study. *British Journal of Addiction*, **83**, 159–70.

Cooke, D. J. and Allan, C. A. (1984). Stressful life events and alcohol abuse in women: a general population study. *British Journal of Addiction*, **79**, 425–30.

Drummond, D. C. (1990). The relationship between alcohol dependence and alcohol-related problems in a clinical population. *British Journal of Addiction*, **85**, 357–66.

Edwards, G. (1986). The alcohol dependence syndrome: concept as stimulus to enquiry. *British Journal of Addiction*, **81**, 171–83.

Edwards, G. and Gross, M. M. (1976). Alcohol dependence: provisional description of a clinical syndrome. *British Medical Journal*, **1**, 1058–61.

Edwards, G., Chandler, J., Hensman, C., and Peto, J. (1972). Drinking in a London Suburb: correlates of trouble with drinking among men. *Quarterly Journal of Studies on Alcohol*, **6**, 94–119.

Edwards, G., Hawker, A., Hensman, C., Peto, J., and Williamson, V. (1973). Alcoholics known or unknown to agencies: epidemiological studies in a London suburb. *British Journal of Psychiatry*, **123**, 169–83.

Edwards, G., Gross, M. M., Keller, M., Moser, J., and Room, R. (1977). Alcohol-related disabilities; WHO Offset Publ. No. 32. Geneva.

Edwards, G., Duckitt, A., Oppenheimer, E., Sheehan, M., and Taylor, C. (1983). What happens to alcoholics? *Lancet*, **2**, 269–71.

Hasin, D. S., Grant, B. F., Harford, T. C., and Endicott, J. (1988). The drug dependence syndrome and related disabilities. *British Journal of Addiction*, **83**, 45–55.

Hesselbrock, V. M., Babor, T. F., Hesselbrock, B., Meyer, R. E., and Workman, K. (1983). 'Never believe an alcoholic?': on the validity of self-report measures of alcohol dependence and related constructs.

Hilton, M. E. (1987*a*). Drinking patterns and drinking problems in 1984: results from a general population survey. *Alcoholism: Clinical and Experimental Research*, **11**, 167–75.

Hilton, M. E. (1987*b*). Demographic characteristics and the frequency of heavy drinking as predictors of self-reported drinking problems. *British Journal of Addiction*, **82**, 913–25.

Hodgson, R. J., Rankin, H. J., and Stockwell, T. (1979). Alcohol dependence and the priming effect. *Behaviour Research and Therapy*, **17**, 379–87.

International Journal of the Addictions, **18**, 593–609.

Jellinek, E. M. (1960). *The disease concept of alcoholism*. Hillhouse, New Brunswick.

Jessor, R. and Jessor, S. L. (1977). *Problem behavior and psychosocial development: a longitudinal study of youth*. Academic Press, New York.

Kenny, D. A. (1979). *Correlation and causality*. Wiley, New York.

Kosten, T. R., Rounsaville, J., Babor, T. F., Spitzer, R. L., and Williams, J. B. W. (1987). Substance use disorders in DSM-III-R: evidence for the dependence syndrome across different psychoactive substances. *British Journal of Psychiatry*, **151**, 834–43.

Langenbucher, J. and Nathan, P. E. (1983). The 'wet' alcoholic: one drink . . . then what? In Cox, W. M. (ed.) *Identifying and measuring Alcoholic personality characteristics*. Jossey Bass, San Fransisco.

Macdonald, S. and Pederson, L. L. (1988). Occurrence and patterns of driving behaviour for alcoholics in treatment. *Drug and Alcohol Dependence*, **22**, 15–25.

Mäkelä, K. and Simpura, J. (1985). Experiences related to drinking as a function of annual intake by sex and age. *Drug and Alcohol Dependence*, **15**, 389–404.

Polich, J. M., Armor, D. J., and Braiker, H. B. (1980). *The course of alcoholism: four years after treatment*. Rand Corporation, Santa Monica.

Rankin, H., Stockwell, T., and Hodgson, R. (1982). Cues for drinking and degree of dependence. *British Journal of Addiction*, **77**, 287–96.

Room, R. (1977). Measurement and distribution of drinking patterns and problems in general populations. In Edwards, G. *et al.* (eds) Alcohol-related disabilities, WHO Offset Publ. No. 32. WHO, Geneva.

Rush, B. (1785). *An enquiry into the effects of spiritous liquors on the human body*. Thomas & Andrews, Boston.

Sadava, S. W. (1985). Problem behavior theory and consumption and consequences of alcohol use. *Journal of Studies on Alcohol*, **46**, 392–7.

Skinner, H. A. (1981). Primary syndromes of alcohol abuse: their measurement and correlates, *British Journal of Addiction*, **76**, 63–76.

Skinner, H. A. (1990). Validation of the dependence syndrome: have we crossed the half-life of this concept? In Edwards G. and Lader M. (eds) *The nature of drug dependence*, Society for the Study of Addiction Monograph No. 1. Oxford University Press, Oxford.

Skinner, H. A. and Goldberg, A. (1986). Evidence for a drug dependence syndrome among narcotic users. *British Journal of Addiction*, **81**, 533–8.

Stockwell, T., Hodgson, R., Edwards, G., Taylor, C., and Rankin, H. (1979). The development of a questionnaire to measure severity of alcohol dependence. *British Journal of Addiction*, **74**, 79–87.

Suppes, P. (1970). A probabilistic theory of causation. North-Holland, Amsterdam.

Trotter, T. (1804). An essay, medical, philosophical, and chemical on drunkenness and its effects on the human body. Longman & Rees, London.

Wanberg, K. W. and Horn, J. L. (1983). Assessment of alcohol use with multidimensional concepts and measures. *American Psychologist*, **38**, 1055–69.

5

Substance-related problems in the context of international classificatory systems

THOMAS F. BABOR

INTRODUCTION

Alcohol and other psychoactive substances engender positive as well as negative consequences for the people who use them, and for society at large. For want of a better term, modern usage of the English language has applied the word 'problem' to the negative consequences of psychoactive substances, and has also personalized the concept by means of terms like 'problem drinker' and 'drug abuser'. The subject of this chapter is less about the nature of these phenomena than about how they are labelled and classified. It begins with a brief history of the classification of substance-related problems in psychiatry and medicine. After reviewing how the nomenclature of substance-related problems has been incorporated into two influential classification systems, the article discusses some broader issues dealing with definitions, and the functions of classification for psychiatry and public health.

NOMENCLATURE, CLASSIFICATION, AND DIAGNOSIS

In psychiatry and medicine, a nomenclature is a list or catalogue of approved terms for describing and recording clinical observations. A nomenclature is necessary for communication among scientists and practitioners working in a field of knowledge, and provides the basis for a classification system. When the names in a nomenclature are grouped together into separate classes, such as mental disorders or substance use disorders, such a grouping is called a classification. The assumptions used to formulate the classes are variable, and depend on the purposes of the classification. In public health and psychiatry, classification of substance use disorders has been conducted according to pharmacological properties, similarity of signs and symptoms, and, to a lesser, extent, the distinction between dependence and substance-related problems.

Diagnosis is the process of identifying and labelling specific disease conditions. The precise attributes used to classify a sick person as having a disease are called diagnostic criteria. The obvious importance of diagnostic criteria and classification systems derives from their usefulness in making clinical decisions, estimating disease prevalence, understanding etiology, and facilitating scientific communication. On a clinical level, diagnostic classification provides a basis for retrieving information about a patient's probable symptoms, the likely course of an illness, and the biological or psychogenic process that underlies the disorder. For example, the *Diagnostic and Statistical Manual* of the American Psychiatric Association is a classification of mental disorders that is based on a systematic description of each disorder in terms of essential features, age of onset, probable course, predisposing factors, associated features, and differential diagnosis. Another purpose of classification is the collection of statistical information on a national and international scale. The International Classification of Diseases (ICD), for example, has as its primary purpose the enumeration of morbidity and mortality data for public health planning. A good classification will also facilitate communication among scientists and provide the basic concepts needed for theory formulation. Both ICD and DSM have been used extensively to classify persons for epidemiological and clinical research. In doing so, classification provides a common frame of reference in communicating scientific findings.

HISTORICAL OVERVIEW

During the nineteenth century there was a great deal of interest in Europe and America in formulating classifications of psychopathology, including substance use disorders (Blashfield 1984; Babor and Lauerman 1986). Up until the early 1800s the classification of mental disorders relating to the use of alcohol and other drugs was crude by current standards, receiving only scant mention in the medical literature.

In the US, the first attempts at classifying alcohol problems are exemplified in the records of nineteenth century asylums, which used such categories as delirium tremens, insanity caused by intemperance, and dipsomania to describe the reasons for a patient's institutionalization. When the condition of chronic drunkenness was 'medicalized' by the early nineteenth century asylum movement, it took the form of a moral–physical concept called intemperance. Later, intemperance was interpreted as a physical and psychological disease that shares many of the same connotations as the current usage of the word alcoholism. Articulated most clearly by Benjamin

Rush (1790) and Samuel Woodward (1838), this early physical disease model of alcoholism became a dominant feature of temperance ideology (Levine 1978). These conceptions assumed an additional dimension favouring psychological causes toward the end of the nineteenth century (Jaffe 1978).

In France, terms like *'folie alcoolique'* and *'ivresse publique'* were part of the standard nomenclature that was used to record morbidity and mortality in the *Annuaire Statistique* throughout the nineteenth century. Other terms that were used in the classification of patients in nineteenth century France included *'buveur d'habitude'* (habitual drinker), *'absinthisme'* (addiction to or consequences of using a toxic mint-flavoured liqueur), and *'buveur d'entrainement'* (socially induced heavy drinking).

In Germany, interest in psychiatric classification culminated with the work of Emil Kraepelin, whose popular textbooks on abnormal psychology became the basis for modern classifications of mental disorders. Although Kraepelin's *Textbook of Psychiatry* (Kraepelin 1909–15) listed intoxication psychoses as one of its 13 major categories, primary emphasis was given to organic disorders associated with chronic alcohol consumption, rather than to less severe manifestations of mental or behavioural problems.

The nosology of drug-related problems is less clear than that of alcohol, having entered the medical nomenclature at the time of the first drug epidemics in the late nineteenth century. The first attempts at classification pertained primarily to opiates and cocaine (Berridge and Edwards 1981). Terms like morphinism and narcomania were used to describe narcotic addiction in the same way that inebriety and dipsomania described alcohol dependence. Other terms used during the late nineteenth century were morphia habit and acute and chronic poisoning by opium.

With the roots of the disease concept firmly planted in nineteenth century medicine and psychiatry, diagnostic classification of substance-related problems up until the 1950s continued to emphasize the concept of addiction, giving lesser attention to the medical, psychological and social problems associated with acute intoxication and chronic substance use.

Thus while most of the attention in the early history of classification systems has clearly been devoted to the more severe manifestations of alcohol- and drug-related disorders, there has also been some consideration given to substance use problems that do not involve addiction or dependence. One example of this can be found in the writings of Jellinek. In his now classic *The Disease Concept of Alcoholism*, Jellinek (1960) proposed five species to account for what he considered to be the most important differences among alcoholics in etiology, natural history, drinking patterns, problems, and prognosis. Jellinek proposed that only when drinking occurs in conjunction with tolerance, withdrawal symptoms, and either loss of control or inability to abstain, should the excessive drinker be termed an 'alcohol addict' and his or her drinking behaviour be regarded as a disease process. Varieties that involved a clear dependence process (gamma and delta types) were contrasted with those that did not (alpha, beta, and epsilon types). The latter types were distinguished primarily by the behavioural, psychological, or social problems that occurred in connection with drinking.

THE INTERNATIONAL CLASSIFICATION OF DISEASES

In its role as the primary international health agency, the World Health Organization (WHO) has played a major role in formulating a nomenclature for the classification of alcohol-related and drug-related disabilities within the International Classification of Diseases (ICD). In the 1950s a series of WHO-sponsored expert committee meetings was convened to discuss issues related to classification and nomenclature (WHO 1952; WHO 1955). Out of these meetings came the first WHO classification of substance-related problems, which was introduced in the eighth edition of ICD under 'Neuroses, personality disorders, and other nonpsychotic mental disorders' (WHO 1967). Here alcoholism (Code 303) was used as a generic category comprised of episodic excessive drinking (dipsomania, periodic drinking bouts), habitual excessive drinking (continual drinking to excess), and alcohol addiction (chronic alcoholism, chronic ethylism). Alcohol addiction in ICD-8 was defined as 'a state of physical and emotional dependence on regular or periodic, heavy, and uncontrolled alcohol consumption, during which the person experiences a compulsion to drink. On cessation of alcohol intake there are withdrawal symptoms, which may be severe' (WHO 1974). What is of equal interest is the allocation of additional categories to excessive drinking, which implies that significant morbidity and mortality may derive from episodic and habitual drinking that does not involve compulsion and withdrawal symptoms.

In the 1974 glossary to ICD-8, episodic excessive drinking was defined as 'relatively brief bouts of excessive consumption of alcohol occurring as frequently as 4 times a year or more. These bouts may last for several days or weeks and may be associated with physical or mental stress or precipitated by cyclical mood changes' (WHO 1974, p. 47). Habitual excessive drinking was defined as 'regular consumption of excessive quantities of alcohol to the detriment of a person's health or social functioning' (WHO 1974, p. 47). It is clear from these definitions that while ICD-8 defined alcoholism broadly at the level of the three-digit codes, it allowed for a more precise distinction between excessive drinking and alcoholic addiction at the level of the four-digit codes.

As indicated in Table 5.1, this distinction was not carried over into the classification of drug dependence (Code 304), which was defined as 'a state, psychic and sometimes also physical, resulting from taking a drug, and characterized by behavioural and other responses that always include a compulsion to take the drug on a continuous or periodic basis in order to experience its psychic effects, and sometimes to avoid the discomfort of its absence' (WHO 1974, pp. 47–48). One possible reason for the lack of a finer distinction between drug dependence and conditions not characterized by dependence in ICD-8 is the fact that in classifications designed primarily for statistical purposes, such as ICD, each section is initially allotted a fixed number of categories. The writers of ICD-8 chose to allocate their ten codes to dependence on specific substances (e.g. opium, synthetic analgesics, etc.) rather than to distinguish between dependence states and other substance use disorders.

Table 5.1 describes the changes in classification that were incorporated into the ninth revision of ICD, which dropped the term alcoholism entirely in favour of alcohol dependence syndrome. This is defined in exactly the same way as drug dependence was in ICD-8 (WHO 1978). Drug dependence maintained the same nomenclature and glossary definition in ICD-9, but a new category was created to accommodate 'Non-dependent abuse of drugs' (Code 305). This category was designed for cases where a person 'has come under medical care because of the maladaptive effect of a drug on which he is not dependent (as defined in Code 304) and that he has taken on his own initiative to the detriment of his health or social functioning' (WHO 1978, pp. 43–4). Because this new three digit abuse category (Code 305) now had ten four digit codes to allocate to different substances, alcohol was listed along with tobacco, cannabis, hallucinogens, barbiturates, tranquillizers, morphine, cocaine, amphetamine, and antidepressants as a possible source of 'non-dependent abuse'. In the case of alcohol, the glossary entry specifies drunkenness, excessive drinking, acute intoxication, 'hangover' effects and inebriety as examples of nondependent abuse.

Although ICD-9 separated alcohol dependence and drug dependence at the level of the three-digit codes, it defined them similarly in terms of a more narrow set of signs and symptoms, and provided an abuse category that included both alcohol and other drugs under the same definition. In doing so ICD made two important assumptions that were to be carried over into ICD-10: (1) that dependence can be classified similarly across a broad range of psychoactive substances; and (2) that substance use in the absence of dependence merits a separate category by virtue of its detrimental effects on health.

During the past decade, the Mental Health Division of WHO has further refined the concept of alcohol and drug dependence to permit classification of different psychoactive substances according to an identical set of criteria

TABLE 5.1 *Classification of substance use disorders in ICD-8, ICD-9, and ICD-10*

ICD-8	ICD-9	ICD-10	
303 Alcoholism	303 Alcohol dependence syndrome	F10–F19	Mental and behavioural disorders due to psychoactive and other substance abuse
303.0 Episodic excessive drinking			
303.1 Habitual excessive drinking	304 Drug dependence		
303.2 Alcohol addiction	304.0 Morphine type		
304 Drug dependence	304.1 Barbiturate type	F10	Disorders resulting from use of alcohol
304.0 Opium, opium alkaloids, and their relatives	304.2 Cocaine		
	304.3 Cannabis	F11	Disorders resulting from use of opioids
	304.4 Amphetamine type and other psychostimulants	F12	Disorders resulting from use of cannabinoids
304.1 Synthetic analgesics with morphine-like effects	304.5 Hallucinogens		
	304.6 Other	F13	Disorders resulting from use of sedatives or hypnotics
304.2 Barbiturates	304.7 Combinations of morphine type drug with any other		
304.3 Other hypnotics and sedatives or tranquillizers			
	304.8 Combinations excluding morphine type drug	F14	Disorders resulting from use of cocaine
304.4 Cocaine			
304.5 Cannabis sativa		F15	Disorders resulting from use of other stimulants (including caffeine)
304.7 Hallucinogenics	304.9 Unspecified		
304.8 Other and combined drugs	305 Non-dependent abuse of drugs		
304.9 Unspecified	305.0 Alcohol	F16	Disorders resulting from use of hallucinogens
	305.1 Tobacco		
	305.2 Cannabis	F17	Disorders resulting from use of tobacco
	305.3 Hallucinogens		
	305.4 Barbiturates and tranquillizers	F18	Disorders resulting from use of volatile solvents
	305.5 Morphine type		
	305.6 Cocaine type	F19	Disorders resulting from multiple drug use and use of other and unidentified substances
	305.7 Amphetamine type		
	305.8 Antidepressants		
	305.9 Other, mixed or unspecified		
		F1x.1*	Harmful use
		F1x.2*	Dependence syndrome
		*4th and 5th character code for specifying the clinical condition.	

in the tenth revision of ICD (WHO 1989; Edwards *et al.* 1976, 1977). A central feature of the ICD-10 approach to substance use disorders is the concept of a dependence syndrome, which is distinguished from disabilities caused by substance use (Edwards *et al.* 1981). The dependence syndrome is defined as an interrelated cluster of psychological symptoms (e.g. a strong desire craving to take the substance), physiological signs (e.g. tolerance and withdrawal), and behavioural indicators (e.g. use of substance to relieve withdrawal discomfort).

Recognizing that many health problems related to alcohol and drug use will be under reported unless appropriate categories are available in the classification system, a WHO memorandum (Edwards *et al.* 1981) and subsequent expert consultations proposed that the term *harmful use* be included in the nomenclature instead of alcohol and drug abuse. The key issue in the definition of this term is the distinction between *perceptions* of adverse effects (e.g. wife complaining about husband's drinking) and actual health consequences (e.g. trauma due to accidents during drug intoxication). Since the purpose of ICD is to classify diseases, injuries, and causes of death, harmful use is defined as a pattern of use which is already causing damage to health. The damage may be either physical (e.g. liver cirrhosis from chronic drinking) or mental (e.g. episodes of depressive disorder secondary to heavy drinking). Harmful patterns of use are often criticized by others and are sometimes associated with adverse social consequences of various kinds. However, the fact that drinking and other substance use are disapproved by the family or culture is not by itself evidence of harmful use.

PSYCHIATRIC CLASSIFICATIONS AND DSM

Although the *Diagnostic and Statistical Manual* of the American Psychiatric Association is not intended to be an international classification system for psychiatric disorders, it has had a major influence on world psychiatry during the past two decades. As discussed below, the third edition of DSM introduced innovations in nomenclature, classification rules, and diagnostic criteria that were adopted with little concern for their cross-cultural applicability by psychiatrists and epidemiologists throughout the world. The remarkable success of DSM is attributable to several factors: its rejuvenation of the Kraepelinian approach to classification, the rich clinical detail it provided, its ready applicability to epidemiological research, and its careful attention to the problem of inter-rater reliability.

The first edition of DSM gave minimal attention to the classification of alcohol and drug disorders. As shown in Table 5.2, the second edition was virtually identical to the alcohol and drug disorders sections of ICD-8. It

TABLE 5.2 Classification of substance use disorders in DSM-II, DSM-III, and DSM-III-R

DSM-II Alcoholism and drug dependence	DSM-III Substance use disorders	DSM-III-R Psychoactive substance use disorders
303.0 Episodic excessive drinking	305.02 Alcohol abuse, episodic	303.90 Alcohol dependence
303.1 Habitual excessive drinking	305.01 Alcohol abuse, continuous	305.00 Alcohol abuse
303.2 Alcohol addiction	303.9x Alcohol dependence	304.40 Amphetamine or similarly acting sympathomimetic dependence
304.0 Drug dependence, opium alkaloids and their derivatives	305.5x Opioid abuse	
	304.0x Opioid dependence	305.70 Amphetamine or similarly acting sympathomimetic abuse
304.1 Drug dependence, synthetic analgesics with morphine-like effects	305.4x Barbiturate or similarly acting sedative or hypnotic abuse	
		304.50 Hallucinogen dependence
304.2 Drug dependence, barbiturates	304.1x Barbiturate or similarly acting sedative or hypnotic dependence	305.30 Hallucinogen abuse
304.3 Drug dependence, other hypnotics and sedatives or 'tranquillizers'		304.60 Inhalant dependence
		305.90 Inhalant abuse
304.4 Drug dependence, cocaine	305.6x Cocaine abuse	305.10 Nicotine dependence
304.5 Drug dependence, Cannabis sativa	305.2x Cannabis abuse	304.00 Opioid dependence
304.6 Drug dependence, other psychostimulants (amphetamines, etc.)	304.3x Cannabis dependence	305.50 Opioid abuse
	305.7x Amphetamine or similarly acting sympathomimetic abuse	304.50 Phencyclidine (PCP) or similarly acting arylcyclohexylamine dependence
	304.4x Amphetamine or similarly acting sympathomimetic dependence	305.90 Phencyclidine (PCP) or similarly acting arylcyclohexylamine abuse
304.7 Drug dependence, hallucinogens	305.9x Hallucinogen abuse	304.10 Sedative, hypnotic, or anxiolytic dependence
	305.9x Phencyclidine (PCP) or similarly acting arylcyclohexylamine	305.40 Sedative, hypnotic, or anxiolytic abuse
	305.1x Tobacco dependence	304.90 Polysubstance dependence
	304.7x Dependence on combination of opioid and other non-alcoholic substance	304.90 Psychoactive substance dependence not otherwise specified
	304.8x Dependence on combination of substances, excluding opioids and alcohol	305.90 Psychoactive substance abuse not otherwise specified

was not until the third edition of DSM that major changes were introduced in the classification of substance use disorders. During the 1970s researchers affiliated with the Washington University School of Medicine (Feighner et al. 1972) began to formulate more reliable diagnostic criteria for the study of alcoholism and other mental disorders in clinical research (Blashfield 1984; Robins 1981; Feighner et al. 1972). This 'research diagnostic' approach strongly influenced the classification of substance use disorders adopted by the American Psychiatric Association (1980) in the third edition of its *Diagnostic and Statistical Manual* (DSM-III). In contrast to previous editions of DSM, alcoholism was now included within the separate category of 'substance use disorders', rather than as a subcategory of personality disorder. Reflecting a trend toward greater semantic precision, the term 'alcohol dependence' was used in preference to the more generic 'alcoholism'. A separate category of 'alcohol abuse' was added to permit greater differentiation, implying that alcohol abuse and alcohol dependence are separate disorders rather than related stages of the same progressive disease process. Alcohol Dependence was distinguished from Alcohol Abuse by the presence of tolerance or withdrawal symptoms. The diagnosis of alcohol abuse included both a pattern of pathological use and impairment in social or occupational functioning due to alcohol.

The definitions of alcohol abuse and dependence in DSM-III made no assumptions about etiology. Rather, DSM-III adopted a behavioural concept of alcohol abuse (pathological use patterns and social impairment) and a bio-behavioural concept of alcohol dependence (tolerance or withdrawal plus a pathological pattern of use).

As part of the American Psychiatric Association's programme of work on diagnostic classification, the entire Substance Use Disorders section of DSM-III was revised in 1987 (Rounsaville et al., 1986; APA, 1987). The most important change involved the adoption of a dimensional model of alcohol and drug dependence that closely resembles the WHO dependence syndrome concept (Edwards et al. 1981). In a significant departure from DSM-III, the medical and social consequences of both acute and chronic intoxication are not among the primary diagnostic criteria of dependence in DSM-III-Revised. These consequences do, however, play a prominent role in the definition of a residual category, substance abuse, which is defined as continued substance use despite persistent social, occupational, psychological, or physical problems that are caused or exacerbated by that substance.

CONCLUSION

The development of nomenclature and classification procedures for alcohol and drug-related problems has been hastened in recent years by practical considerations: the need for better communication among clinicians, researchers, and international health agencies; the need for decision rules to categorize people with substance use disorders for epidemiological, medical, or psychiatric reasons; and the need for diagnostic tools in planning treatment.

What is evident from this review is that diagnostic criteria, nomenclature, and classification rules for substance use disorders have undergone substantial evolution during the past century. Initially, definitions focused on either the consequences of chronic substance use or the more specific process of addiction. In the latter part of the nineteenth century and the early decades of the twentieth, greater attention was given to the etiological basis of the disorder, especially in terms of the pharmacology of dependence. During the latter half of the twentieth century there has been a continued effort to define the place of problems in classification of diseases and disorders. The medical model, based on the assumption that alcoholism and addiction are distinct disease entities having physical manifestations, has been gradually supplanted by a concept that views dependence as a behavioural and psychiatric disorder that is conceptually distinct from the medical, psychological, and social problems that often are associated with it.

Recent work on the revision of two influential diagnostic systems (ICD and DSM), used extensively for the classification of substance use disorders, has led to a synthesis of the two approaches. Both systems now define alcohol dependence according to the elements first proposed by Edwards and Gross (1976). Both systems now also include a residual category (harmful alcohol use [ICD]; alcohol abuse [DSM]) that allows classification of psychological and medical consequences directly related to the ingestion of alcohol, when these are associated with a regular pattern of use. Finally, both systems have adopted similar criteria for the classification of disorders connected with all psychoactive substances, implying that the similarities across substances are greater than the differences.

Implicit in these revisions is a model of substance-related problems that considers harmful consequences and dependence symptoms as independent but potentially interrelated diagnostic categories.

Drug and alcohol use are associated with a wide variety of psychological, social, and medical problems that result from the direct effects of intoxication (e.g. accidents, aggressive behaviour), the sequelae of intoxication (e.g. depression, delusional symptoms), or the cumulative effects of chronic substance use (e.g. liver disease, insomnia, paranoid thinking). Problems that occur in the absence of dependence are rated somewhat differently in DSM and ICD. Table 5.3 summarizes the criteria used to diagnose harmful alcohol use in ICD-10 and alcohol abuse in DSM-III-R. These residual categories permit the classification of maladaptive patterns of use that do

TABLE 5.3 *ICD-10 and DSM-III-R diagnostic criteria for harmful alcohol use and alcohol abuse*

Nature of Criteria	ICD-10 Criteria for harmful use	DSM-III-R Criteria for alcohol abuse
Symptom criteria	Clear evidence that alcohol use is responsible for causing actual psychological or physical harm to the user.	A maladaptive pattern of alcohol use indicated by at least one of the following: (1) continued use despite knowledge of having a persistent or recurrent social, occupational, psychological, or physical problem that is caused or exacerbated by alcohol use; or (2) recurrent use in situations in which alcohol use is physically hazardous (e.g. driving while intoxicated).
Duration criterion	The pattern of use has persisted for at least 1 month or has occurred repeatedly over the previous 12 months.	Some symptoms of the disturbance have persisted for at least 1 month, or have occurred repeatedly over a longer period of time.

not meet criteria for alcohol dependence. The diagnoses of abuse or harmful use are designed primarily for drinkers or drug users who have recently begun to experience substance-related problems, and for chronic users whose consequences develop in the absence of marked dependence symptoms. Examples of situations in which these categories would be appropriate include: (1) a pregnant woman who keeps using alcohol even though her physician has told her that it could be responsible for fetal damage; (2) a college student whose weekend marijuana smoking results in missed classes, poor grades, and traffic accidents; and (3) a middle-aged beer drinker who develops high blood pressure and fatty liver in the absence of alcohol dependence symptoms.

While recognizing that adverse social consequences often accompany substance use, social problems in ICD-10 are not in themselves sufficient to result in a diagnosis of 'harmful use'. As noted in the ICD diagnostic guidelines (WHO 1989), harmful patterns of substance use are often criticized by others and sometimes are legally prohibited by governments. The fact that drinking is disapproved by another person or by the drinker's culture is not in itself evidence of harmful use, unless socially negative consequences have actually occurred at dosage levels that also result in psychological and physical consequences. This is a major difference that distinguishes ICD-10s harmful use from DSM-III-Rs alcohol abuse. The latter category permits the use of social consequences in the diagnosis of abuse.

Another difference between harmful use and alcohol abuse is that the latter includes recurrent use in situations that are physically hazardous, such as driving a car or caring for children. This means that alcohol abuse is likely to be much more prevalent than harmful use, in part because of the hazardous use criterion, and in part because of the incorporation of social consequences into the DSM-III-R criteria.

An important conceptual and theoretical issue is whether dependence is sufficiently distinct from abuse or harmful use to be considered a separate condition. In DSM-III-R, substance abuse is a residual category that allows the clinician to classify clinically meaningful aspects of a patient's behaviour when that behaviour is not clearly associated with a dependence syndrome (Rounsaville *et al.*, 1986). In ICD-10, harmful use implies identifiable medical or psychiatric consequences that occur in the absence of a dependence syndrome. In both classification systems, dependence is conceived as an underlying condition that has much greater clinical significance, primarily because of its implications for understanding etiology, predicting course, and planning treatment.

The present conceptualization of harmful use and substance abuse makes assumptions about the association between problem behaviour and personal characteristics other than substance use. Substance-related problems are often associated with a variety of personal and social antecedents that can increase vulnerability to substance-related problems. For example, certain population groups (e.g. persons who are older, female, and low in body mass) are more vulnerable to the acute effects of intoxication than are other population groups (e.g. younger males who are overweight). Similarly, there may be personality characteristics, such as sociopathy, that predispose some people to act aggressively while using substances like cocaine or phencyclidine (PCP), or biological characteristics that predispose some drinkers to develop cirrhosis or pancreatitis. Social antecedents may also be considered vulnerability factors. Socially learned attitudes may lead a drinker to expect that alcohol will 'cause' the release of aggression or sexual inhibitions, and he or she may act in accordance with these expectations regardless of the pharmacological effects of ethanol. Social norms that tolerate excessive drinking, as in France; or which call for punishing drunkenness as in Islamic societies, may result in drastically different consequences for the drinker. Socially-learned drinking customs, like buying rounds or toasting to one's health, may predispose large segments of the male population in a country like France or the Soviet Union to drink intensively in response to social pressures. These should be taken into account in the diagnosis of harmful use.

Alternative approaches to substance-related problems, promulgated largely by more quantitatively oriented social and behavioural scientists, have been proposed as if the so-called medical model precluded consideration of a non-disease classification. For example, behavioural approaches to the definition of alcoholism have been advanced in recent years (Nathan 1981; Pattison *et al.* 1977) as alternatives to what has come to be called the 'traditional disease concept', i.e. the notion that alcoholism is a unitary disease entity having a prescribed etiology from physical or psychological causes, as well as a coherent pattern of signs and symptoms. These approaches reject binary classification and make few, if any, assumptions about the biological or psychogenic basis of the underlying disorder. Emphasis is given instead to the observable behaviour of the drinker, how that behaviour is learned and modified by antecedent conditions and reinforcing consequences, and the problems resulting from the act of drinking.

Since cultural context is an important determinant of substance use patterns and consequences, an organizing principle which has cross-cultural applicability is very desirable. A focus on psychobiological 'universals' in the face of cultural diversity offers promise for a more widely applicable classification system. Social consequences reduce the cross-cultural applicability of diagnostic criteria. For example, changes in legal definitions, controls, or mandates in different countries will markedly influence the relationship between substance use and legal consequences. Hence, having a substance use disorder will be more heavily influenced by specific cultural mores within DSM than in ICD.

There is an important conceptual distinction between the underlying condition driving substance abuse (dependence), and the consequences of substance use. Legal and medical consequences often result from acute intoxication rather than dependence *per se*. Social and psychological consequences are sometimes more a function of pre-existing or co-morbid psychiatric disorders than of an underlying dependence syndrome. Although there have been important modifications in the classification of substance use disorders during the past three decades, the fundamental distinction between dependence and harmful use has been maintained with remarkable consistency throughout the modern history of classification.

REFERENCES

American Psychiatric Association (1980). *Diagnostic and statistical manual of mental disorders* (3rd edn). Washington, DC.

American Psychiatric Association (1987). *Diagnostic and statistical manual of mental disorders* (3rd edn, revised). Washington, DC.

Babor, T. F. and Lauerman, R. (1986). Classification and forms of inebriety: Historical antecedents of alcohol typologies. In Galanter, M. (ed), *Recent Developments in Alcoholism*, Vol. V, pp. 113–44, Plenum Press, New York.

Berridge, V. and Edwards, G. (1981). *Opium and the people*. Allen Lane/St. Martin's Press, London/New York.

Blashfield, R. K. (1984). *The classification of psychopathology.* Plenum Press, New York.
Edwards, G. and Gross, M. M. (1976). Alcohol dependence: Provisional description of a clinical syndrome. *British Medical Journal,* 1, 1058–61.
Edwards, G., Gross, M. M., Keller, M., and Moser, J. (eds) (1976). Alcohol-related problems in the disability perspective. *Journal of Studies on Alcohol,* 37, 1360–82.
Edwards, G., Gross, M. M., Keller, M. Moser, J., and Room, R. (eds) (1977). *Alcohol-related disabilities,* WHO Offset Publ. No. 32. WHO Geneva.
Edwards, G., Arif, A., and Hodgson, R. (1981). Nomenclature and classification of drug-and alcohol-related problems: a WHO memorandum. *Bulletin of the World Health Organization,* 59(2), 225–42.
Feighner, J., Robins, E., Guze, S., Woodruff, R., Winokur, G., and Munoz, R. (1972). Diagnostic criteria for in psychiatric research. *Archives of General Psychiatry,* 26, 57–63.
Jaffe, A. (1978). Reform in American medical science: the inebriety movement and the origins of the psychological disease theory of addiction, 1870–1920. *British Journal of Addiction,* 73, 139–47.
Jellinek, E. M. (1960). *The disease concept of alcoholism.* Hillhouse, New Brunswick.
Kraepelin, E. (1909–1915). *Psychiatrie: ein Lehrbuch* (8th edn), 4 vols. J. A. Barth, Leipzig, Germany.
Levine, H. G. (1978). The discovery of addiction: changing conceptions of habitual drunkenness in America. *Journal of Studies on Alcohol,* 39, 143–74.
Nathan, P. E. (1981). Prospects for a behavioral approach to the diagnosis of alcoholism. In Meyer, R. E., Babor, T. F., Glueck, B. C., Jaffe, J. H., O'Brien, J. E., and Stabenau, J. R. (eds) *Evaluation of the alcoholic: implications for research, theory and treatment* NIAAA Research Monograph #5, DHHS Publication No. (ADM) 81–1033, pp. 85–102, Washington, DC.
Pattison, E. M., Sobell, M. B., and Sobell, L. C. (1977). *Emerging concepts of alcohol dependence.* Springer, New York.
Robins, L. (1981). The diagnosis of alcoholism after DSM III. In Meyer, R. E., Babor, T. F., Glueck, B. C., Jaffe, J. H., O'Brien, J. E., and Stabenau, J. R. (eds) *Evaluation of the alcoholic: implications for research, theory and treatment.* NIAAA Research Monograph #5, DHHS Publication No. (ADM) 81–1033, pp. 85–102, Washington, DC.
Room, R. (1983). Sociological aspects of the disease concept of alcoholism. In Smart, R. G., Glaser, F. B., Israel, Y., Kalant, H., Popham, R. E., and Schmidt W. (eds), *Research Advances in Alcohol and Drug Problems,* Vol. 7, Plenum Press, New York, pp. 47–92.
Rounsaville, B. J., Spitzer, R. L., and Williams, J. B. W. (1986). Proposed changes in the DSM-III substance use disorders: description and rationale. *American Journal of Psychiatry.* 143, 463–8.
Rush, B. (1790). *An inquiry into the effects of spirituous liquors on the human body.* Thomas & Andrews, Boston.
Spitzer, R. L., Endicott, J., and Robins, E. (1975). *Research diagnostic criteria (RDC) for a selected group of functional disorders.* New York State Psychiatric Institute, New York.

Woodward, S. B. (1838). *Essays on asylums for inebriates*. Worcester Asylum, Worcester, Massachusetts.
World Health Organization (1952). *Expert committee on mental health, alcoholism subcommittee, Second Report*. Technical Report Series No. 48. WHO, Geneva.
World Health Organization (1955). *Alcohol and Alcoholism, report of an expert Committee*. Technical Report Series No. 94. WHO, Geneva.
World Health Organization (1967). Manual of the International Classification of Diseases, Injuries, and Causes of Death (1965 revision). WHO, Geneva.
World Health Organization (1974). *Glossary of mental disorders and guide to their classification: for use in conjunction with the international Classification of Diseases* (8th revision). WHO, Geneva.
World Health Organization (1978). *Mental disorders: glossary and guide to their classification in accordance with the ninth revision of the international classification of diseases*. WHO, Geneva.
World Health Organization (1989). *International classification of diseases*, (10th revision) 1989. Draft of Chapter V: Mental, behavioural and developmental disorders: clinical descriptions and diagnostic guidelines. WHO, Geneva.

6

Drinking problems: the individual in social context

NORMAN KREITMAN

This chapter will take the individual-in-context as the object of study. This, the author believes, is what distinguishes modern epidemiology from other more piecemeal approaches. The distinction between population and individual considerations relates only to levels and types of data. It is on this premise that most of the following observations are organized. First, however, it is necessary to say something about the concept of misuse and the specification of problems.

THE CONCEPT OF 'MISUSE'

'Substance misuse' is a term which carries two implications. The first is that 'misuse' is something other than 'use', and second, that misuse can be distinguished by being associated with consequences which are in some sense undesirable.

Each of these rather obvious points raises difficulties, which may vary somewhat according to the substance in question. Thus in our society, marijuana is officially viewed as a substance which is innately harmful, so that possession of the drug and trafficking in it are proscribed by law. (Consumption *per se* is not illegal in the UK but this is only because of difficulties of proof.) Alcohol, on the other hand, is in many cultures not seen as intrinsically undesirable. Elsewhere in this book, Harry Levine has elegantly demonstrated how such views — on beverage alcohol itself as distinct from its effects — change in different historical periods, while in the contemporary world one need only point to teetotal communities where *any* consumption of alcohol is stigmatized. Similarly, in the WHO Three Nation Study (Ritson 1985), it was found that Mexican, but not Scottish or Zambian wives, typically condemned any alcohol consumption by their husbands, rather than confining their complaint to specific intoxicated behaviour.

However, this issue is less pervasive than the second, concerning the specification of what constitutes a 'problem' in a drug consuming society. (The following discussion is centred on alcohol, but could also apply to other drugs.) Here the student is at once confronted by cultural relativity, operating both between different societies and between segments of the same community. The relevant literature is very extensive, and can scarcely be summarized. It appears that investigators have in practice identified up to three separate sources for the designation of behaviours as 'problematic'. There is first the consumer of the substance, declaring what he or she regards as a problem; these may cover any aspect of physical or mental health, or of social function. Most surveys, for example, use self-report as the primary means of problem identification though recognizing that when communicating with the interviewer, consumers take a highly conservative view of their problems in comparison to the accounts of others. Note that although problems elicited directly from respondents tend to be seen as individual attributes, many of the problems so identified are in fact interactive with the social environment (such as marital quarrels), rather than being purely personal (like hepatic impairment).

The second identifying agent is the social group around the individual — family, employer, or society at large. Such agents declare a given item to be undesirable from their point of view whatever that may be. Their justification for adverse judgements are not at issue although of considerable interest in their own right.

The third agent — and this is sometimes overlooked — is that of the qualified observer. Thus Knupfer (1972) states:

If a person chooses to spend a lot of his time in a state of intoxication, who is to say that that is a problem? My position is that if either he thinks it is a problem or his wife does, or his boss does, or he gets arrested for drunkenness, then it is a problem, *I also reserve the right to decide that it is a problem*, even without those conditions, if he drinks, say, a fifth of whisky a day.
(Italics added)

This — to risk a pun — is a highly fluid definition, but it serves to emphasize that pathological changes may, in medical terms, be detected at the pre-symptomatic stage and must surely feature among the undesirable consequences of drinking.

We require then to accept that problems may be defined from any or all of these three viewpoints. Each should be distinguished and each allowed equal legitimacy without premature concern for the social values which doubtless underpin them. But the interesting question is how and why a problem, however identified, is generated. The approach which my own group has found helpful entails the recognition that a number of moderating factors intervene between the ingestion of a given quantity of the substance and any subsequent change. These include, for example, body mass, sexually-differentiated metabolic pathways, personality, and the social context, and are mentioned here solely for completeness. Arbitrarily, it takes consumption as the starting point of the process, if only because a research programme has to delimit its range; one has to start somewhere. The model is:

```
Consumption – – ┬ – – Consequences – – ┬ – – Problems (as defined by
               |                       |                    – self
            Mediators                Context                – others/agencies
                                                            – observer)
```

The model as set out is more elaborate than is required for *all* consequences, such as those relating to impairment of physical health and the development of the alcohol-dependence syndrome. It seems very reasonable to assume that anyone whose health is significantly damaged, or who has developed the physical and psychological symptoms of dependence, can be considered to be in a state of distress and hence to have a problem. Considerable caution is however required in assuming that the process ends at that point when we are considering, for example, alcohol intoxication, or disruption in the social, marital and public order areas. To take the first of these, a state of moderate inebriation is not necessarily problematic, and to declare it so in advance of evidence is to close the door on the possibilities of analysis. Some illustrative findings will be given below.

THE PROBLEM OF ASCRIPTION

An important issue arises when an attempt is made to specify a 'problem' in operational terms, even after the conceptual issues have been more or less clarified. The difficulty here is the so called problem of ascription, a topic which has been inadequately considered in the literature.

Let us suppose that preliminary evidence exists for an association between consumption of a drug, say alcohol, and some item of behaviour such as being arrested by the police. The next step in an inquiry is likely to be an attempt to specify the magnitude of the association in a given society. For this we would require to specify, with respect to a defined period, how many individuals had been drinking and how many had been arrested, recognising that of course each of these can occur without the other. But this is not sufficient; in some sections of society both drinking and being arrested are common, and coincidence can occur by chance or come about only very indirectly. It is, in other words, necessary to make explicit our implicit interest, which is how often arrests can be ascribed to alcohol. Exactly the same kinds of questions arise in connection with physical health, marital conflict, impaired working efficiency, and so forth.

The ascription of a given behaviour or illness to alcohol may be quite difficult if the behaviour in question is multifactorial in origin, as is so commonly the case. In a survey, for example, it becomes necessary for the interviewer carefully to probe the respondent's report to ascertain whether, for the example concerning police arrests, there was any temporal association between the behaviour and drinking, whether and how often some of the behaviours occur during phases of sobriety, whether the respondent himself or others ascribed the behaviour and so on. A quasi-clinical style of questioning is required, but standard list of prompts can however be very useful and can make a major difference to the results. Thus in one of our studies, which will be cited again later, a group of factory workers admitted to a total of 247 instances of work-related behaviours of a kind which had been postulated a priori as possibly linked to alcohol, such as Monday morning absenteeism or a progressive decline in work standards. Of these only 77 were finally accepted as being so; the remainder were due to other causes such as physical illhealth not obviously related to alcohol.

AGGREGATE VS INDIVIDUAL DATA

We may now pass on to consider the types of data which may be employed in studies of how problems are generated, and to review the way in which epidemiological techniques may be used as a basic science (rather than in estimating service needs, etc), in understanding the processes. It will be argued that the essential difference between the two main epidemiological approaches, the aggregate and the individual, lies in the number of variables which can be measured simultaneously with respect to each individual in a study population.

The term aggregate data is used to refer to information which concerns a population as a whole, but where little if any specification is possible of which individuals in the group carry the phenomena of interest. More formally, aggregate data are an array in which it is not possible to specify each individual in terms of all the classificatory variables simultaneously, or alternatively it is one in which individuals cannot be cross-classified in terms of the main axes. An example might be a population described in terms of the rates for some disorder for males and females, and separately by age, but with no information on the rate for young men, old women, etc. This limitation is absolutely basic, and cannot be circumvented by considering a series of communities. If a number of cities are ranked by, say, alcohol consumption and again by their rates for traffic accidents, then a positive rank order correlation is *not* evidence that accidents are due to

Drinking problems in social context   103

TABLE 6.1 *Associations at the ecological and individual level*

(a)	At ecological level	% Illiterate	% Migrants
	Town A	10	20
	Town B	20	30
	Town C	30	40

(b)	At individual level		Illiterate	
			Yes	No
	Town A			
	Migrant	Yes	0	200
		No	100	700
	Town B			
	Migrant	Yes	0	300
		No	200	500
	Town C			
	Migrant	Yes	0	400
		No	300	300

There is perfect ecological concordance between illiteracy and migration, yet not a single migrant is illiterate in any of the three towns. Within each town the two variables are negatively related.

drinking. The use of discrete communities in this way as though they were single individuals was recognized as the so-called ecological fallacy at least as early as 1950 when it was pointed out by Robinson. Table 6.1 illustrates that in a hypothetical situation a series of communities may be perfectly and positively correlated in their rates for two characteristics, and yet for each of them to show a *negative* correlation between the variables when considered at an individual level.

It must be added that later authors (e.g. Hanushek *et al.* 1974; Firehaugh 1978) have challenged Robinson's analysis, and have proposed to salvage the legitimacy of the ecological approach to causal analysis at the individual level. These arguments have so far failed to persuade epidemiologists to abandon their deep-seated suspicion of the method when applied outside certain very limited contexts.

It should also be noted in defence of aggregate data that *inter alia* they may be used for predictive purposes once a direct link between the variables of interest has been already established (Morgenstern 1982). Thus trends in alcohol consumption will point to the likely frequency of liver cirrhosis. In this instance the converse prediction is more often made, namely from known levels of liver cirrhosis to the consumption habits of the population. The most interesting use of aggregate data, however, is when they are used to characterize communities and to raise questions concerning social structures and processes. In Edinburgh, areas of the city with high rates of *male* unemployment have been found to have high rates of *female* parasuicide. Different individuals contribute to the numerators of the two kinds of rate, but each is a reflection of a common underlying factor, namely familial disorganization. Investigations along such lines are of course of great interest, and it is important not to regard aggregate data as somehow 'second class'. The essential point is that individual-level and aggregate data are qualitatively different; both have their value but their proper uses should not be confused.

INDIVIDUAL LEVEL DATA

For practical purposes the only method to obtain information by which to characterize individuals in terms of a number of variables is by the epidemiological survey. These are expensive to mount, laborious to carry out, and exhausting to analyse. They are not to be undertaken lightly, but the survey does provide the route to examining the interaction of multiple factors judged likely to be relevant.

Some examples in relation to the kind of model previously discussed may help at this point. The first is from an early study conducted in San Francisco in 1964 (Knupfer 1967). One of the interests of that study was to determine whether, (i) gender and (ii) socio-economic status mediated the relationship between level of alcohol consumption and the adverse social consequences of heavy drinking. Table 6.2 shows that the answer to the first question is no, and to the second yes. Given frequent high intake the risks of suffering adverse social effects were approximately the same in men and women but increased steeply from the highest to the lowest socio-economic group, among both sexes.

A similar example is from the US national survey reported by Cahalan and Room (1974). They investigated the same kind of question but with respect to a wider range of possible moderating variables. Table 6.3 summarizes some of the results and shows that among heavy drinkers the proportion suffering from adverse effects, as defined in the study, varied by each of the four moderator variables listed. Of these the local drinking culture seemed to be the most important.

Lastly, we may refer back to the formal model set out earlier in this paper. It was tested in a small survey which covered men drawn selectively from high and low social status groups, since social class was of particular interest to us at that time. As with the two previous studies, level of consumption was taken as the primary axis. Among other things, we asked whether intake was related to having one or more of the symptoms of the alcohol dependence syndrome as described by Edwards and Gross (1976). Figure 6.1 illustrates that there was no difference whatsoever between the

TABLE 6.2 *High consumption and adverse social effects in San Francisco: 1964*

	(a) Freqent high intake (%)	(b) Adverse social effects (%)*	(b) as % of (a)
Sex:			
Males (N = 426)	29	8	27
Female (N = 544)	9	2	22
Socio-economic status:			
High (N = 103)	23	1	4
Middle (N = 427)	19	4	21
Low (N = 359)	16	6	37
	From Knupfer (1967)		

* The original report designates this column as 'serious social consequences'.

TABLE 6.3 *Heavy intake and adverse consequences: USA 1967–1969*

	(N)	(a) Heavy intake: no adverse consequences (%)	(b) Heavy intake + adverse consequences (%)	$\frac{(b)}{(a)+(b)}$ (%)
Age				
21–4	(147)	16	31	66
25+	(1414)	12	12	50
Residence				
Dry region	(652)	8	15	65
Wet region	(909)	15	13	46
Upbringing				
Rural, towns	(913)	9	14	61
Cities	(467)	17	14	45
Social class				
Lowest	(281)	14	26	65
Others	(1280)	12	11	49
		From Cahalan and Room (1974)		

two groups, and that both showed a curvilinear relationship between consumption and the presence of symptoms. We similarly failed to find within each group any effect for a range of other mediators — including drinking style, age, social class of origin, and many others — with respect to any evidence of alcohol dependence. (However, if the dependent variable was

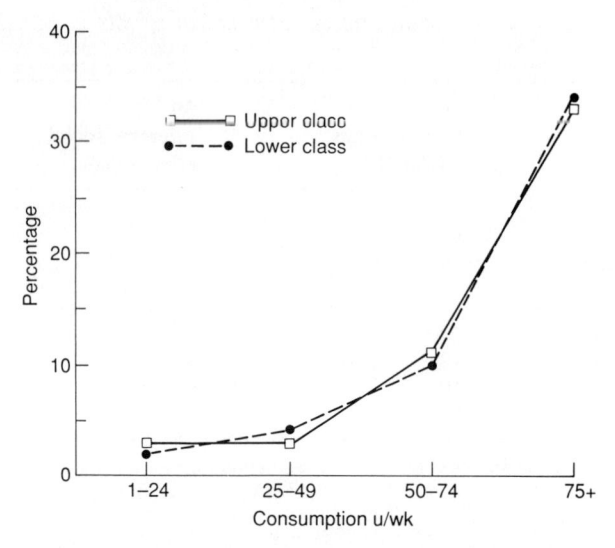

FIG. 6.1 Consumption and alcohol dependence syndrome, by social group.

defined as *severity* of alcohol dependence, clear differences did emerge between the social classes. Thus at weekly consumption levels of 50–74 units of alcohol, the lower class group reported mean scores on a scale of alcohol dependence at twice the level of the upper social class group.) There was however, evidence for the role of contextual variables with respect to certain other consequences of drinking and whether they were 'problematic'. Work impairment was one example. Figure 6.2 shows that at given levels of consumption, the lower social class group was much more likely to experience work-related consequences that the upper class group. (The explanations probably include aspects of drinking style and the externally-imposed rigidity of the working environment of the lower class group.)

But it was possible to go further with the question of why only some individuals whose drinking affected their work found this to be a 'problem'. Each group was analysed separately. Thus among the upper class respondents, 31, representing 11 per cent of the sample, admitted to some degree of alcohol-related impairment of work performance. Of these only about half considered this a problem (15/31, 48 per cent) and these men were found to be (a) older and (b) to have wives who were critical of their drinking habits. Thus in a descriptive sense both these variables act as contextual variables in terms of the model on p. 101. Of course the interpretation of the finding requires further exploration — we tested three or four possibilities ourselves and doubtless others could be advanced. Inter-

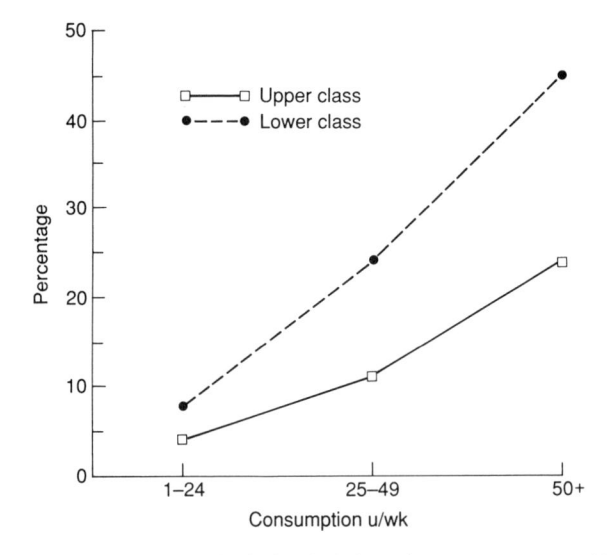

FIG. 6.2 Consumption and alcohol-related work consequences (1+) by social group.

estingly these contextual variables did not operate in the same way in the lower class sample. It seems that the factors which turn the behavioural consequences of drinking into problems, may be quite subtle and may operate differently in different segments of society.

These comments and examples are intended to argue the case for a way of thinking about alcohol problems, and a strategy for data analysis. It is evident that it is only feasible given detailed individually-based data such as surveys can provide.

MODELS AND THEORIES

Finally it may be salutory to remind ourselves that a statistical model is no more than a working tool for investigating a theory. It is all too easy to lose sight of that connection. Interest can easily switch to modifying the statistical model, by determining, for example, whether certain variables do or do not act as mediators in certain types of relationship, and to forget that we are in fact dealing with a substantive process operating in the real world. Debates about the subtleties of logistic linear regression and the like are important but only as precursors to hard thought about the biological, pharmacological, and sociological aspects of problem drinking.

REFERENCES

Cahalan, D. and Room, R. (1974). *Problem drinking among American men Rutgers Center for Alcohol Studies*, Monograph Series No. 7. New Brunswick, New Jersey.

Edwards, G. and Gross, M. (1976). Alcohol dependence: provisional description of a clinical syndrome. *British Medical Journal*, **1**, 1058–61.

Firehaugh, G. (1978). A rule of inferring individual level relationships from aggregate data. *American Sociological Review*, **43**, 557–72.

Hanushek, E., Jackson, J., and Kain J. (1974). Model specification, use of aggregate data and the ecological correlation fallacy. *Political Methodology*, **1**, 89–107.

Knupfer, G. (1967). The epidemiology of problem drinking. *American Journal of Public Health*, **57**, 973–86.

Knupfer, G. (1972). Ex-problem Drinkers. In Roff, M., Robins, L. N., and Pollock M. (eds) *Life History Research in Psychopathology*, Vol 2. University of Minnesota Press, Minneapolis.

Morgenstern, H. (1982). Uses of ecological analysis in epidemiological research. *American Journal of Public Health*, **72**, 1336–44.

Ritson, E. B. (1985). *Community response to alcohol related problems*. Public Health Paper 81. WHO, Geneva.

Robinson, W. (1950). Ecological correlations and the behaviour of individuals. *American Sociological Review*, **15**, 351–7.

7

The role of culture in the drug question

GEOFFREY PEARSON

The notion of 'culture' is invoked in many different ways in public discourses on drug problems. At one extreme, it is said that we live in a 'drug dependent culture'. At the other, that the values of our culture are threatened by drugs. The term 'drug culture', particularly applied to the young, has entered into our everyday language. An important area of scientific concern is the extent to which cultural factors mediate and influence the pharmacological effects of drugs.

The argument developed here will proceed by a series of examples, which although by no means exhaustive will indicate the ways in which the question of culture is addressed within the field of drug use and misuse. This exploratory, step-by-step approach, while it will not deliver a clear-cut conclusion, will nevertheless attempt to clarify the terms of the debate. The first step in this clarificatory process must be what we mean by 'culture'.

THE MEANINGS OF CULTURE

'Culture', according to Raymond Williams (1983) in his *Keywords*, 'is one of the two or three most complicated words in the English language'. He continues:

This is so partly because of its intricate historical development, in several European languages, but mainly because it has now come to be used for important concepts in several distinct intellectual disciplines and in several distinct and incompatible systems of thought.

It is beyond the scope of this paper to rehearse the entire history of the word, which involves several decisive shifts of meaning. It begins in English as a noun describing the process of tending crops and animals, leading to what is at first a metaphorical application to human affairs: for example, 'the culture and manurance of minds' by Bacon in 1605. It is in this sense that it becomes associated with 'cultivated' manners or a 'cultured' mind. In the eighteenth century, the word passed through a series of transformations principally in the German language, to emerge as a term meaning 'civilization' and hence the varying 'cultures' of different nations and historical periods. The notion of 'folk culture' or 'folklore', which first appears in English in 1846, involves a further transformation in the context of the urban and industrial revolutions, to indicate a 'popular culture' or 'tradition' which is being lost within the experience of modernity (Pearson 1985). Through social anthropology this emphasis is subsequently developed, as in the title of Tylor's *Primitive Culture* (1871), whereby culture comes to mean a 'whole way of life'. Later, through sociology, we arrive at 'subculture' to represent the culture of a distinguishable smaller group — as in 'youth culture' or 'drug culture'.

This summary of the word's complex development allows us to distinguish three broad approaches around which this paper will be organized. First, the idea of culture as a 'whole way of life' and the exploration of variations in drug practices within the perspective of cultural relativism. Second, research on particular drug subcultures and the lifestyles associated with drug use. Finally, culture as a 'cultivation of habits' or 'socialization', where attention is given to the ways in which culture confers social meanings to drug practices, both in the sense of mediating the pharmacological effects of drugs and also socializing drug users into specific ways of using and understanding drugs.

CULTURE AS A 'WHOLE WAY OF LIFE': CULTURAL RELATIVISM

At the most general level, reflecting the profound tendency of social anthropology to see things in relative terms, we might begin by asking in what ways different cultures define what is meant by 'drugs' and 'drug misuse'. The inclination to employ some form of intoxicant is a near-universal across the otherwise intricate twists and turns of human conduct revealed by social anthropology. Even so, different cultures adopt different lines of demarcation as to what are to be understood as acceptable or unacceptable forms of drug-taking.

It is, for example, something of a jolt to learn that in nineteenth century India opium 'remained the ordinary Indian's remedy for malaria, his rejuvenator in old age, the agent of his relief from fatigue and pain — no more to be frowned upon than bhang or hashish' (Fay 1976). A retired Indian civil servant, giving evidence before the Royal Commission on Opium in 1893, thought that 'the best practical answer to those who inveigh against the use of opium would be, if such a thing were practicable, to bring one of our crack opium-drinking Sikh regiments to London and exhibit them in Hyde Park' (quoted in Fay 1976). It was opium-eating which was tolerated in the Indian subcontinent, while opium-smoking was less well known, and even frowned upon.

Through historical research both in Britain and North America, we have become familiar with the large measure of tolerance shown towards both opiates and cocaine preparations in our own societies in the nineteenth century (Musto 1973; Berridge & Edwards 1981). Suffice to say that cultural relativism indicates the need for a comparative understanding of drug use and the definition of drug problems, both in terms of cross-cultural studies and also through historical time within any given culture.

Originally, cultural variations in drug use would have been decisively influenced by climate, the fertility of land, and other circumstances bearing upon local variations in plant life. Tobacco is an obvious case, widely used by Amerindians, but unknown in Europe until it was encountered by Columbus in the 'New World' (Wilbert 1987). On the other hand, the ubiquitous chemistry of fermentation means that alcoholic beverages were almost universally known, although not always approved. Even within the same geographical terrain, moreover, cultural variations — in terms of, for example, religion, status, caste — might mean that different social groups would select from the repertoire of available intoxicants, embracing one while rejecting another. An instance of this type of local cultural variation was found in the study by Carstairs (1954), of the differential use of bhang and alcohol by the two highest caste groups (Rajput and Brahmin) in a village in Rajasthan. For the warrior-like Rajput, alcohol was the preferred drug, whereas for the Brahmins it was utterly rejected. Nevertheless, cannabis intoxication was commonplace among even the most holy Brahmins:

Again and again the writer was able to see respectable Brahmins and holy *Saddhus* who were benignly and conspicuously fuddled with bhang. To his eye, they were drunk as lords — drunk as Rajputs — and yet they would have been mortally offended if the comparison had been drawn, because this form of intoxication they believed not only no disgrace, but actually an enhancement of the spiritual life.

In the course of the late nineteenth and early twentieth centuries, the vast expansion of commerce laid the basis for the universal spread of virtually all known drugs. Whereupon, it was local systems of morality and legal regulation which came to define the main contours of the cultural diversity of accepted drug practices. If culture is defined as a 'whole way of life', then that way of life will include the systems of legal regulation which have come to surround drug use.

Law as an aspect of culture

Such an approach lends itself to the strongest form of argument that culture determines drug problems: in the sense that culture, through its systems of legal regulation, most emphatically defines what is a 'drug problem' and what is not, with sometimes surprising results. We need only reflect on our own culture's tolerance of alcohol and tobacco use, with their damaging consequences for personal and public health, to grasp the relevance of cultural relativism.

An associated question is whether specific forms of legal regulation, in themselves, amplify the problem of drug misuse. In a nutshell, does the criminalization of drugs increase 'secondary' effects such as drug-related crime, trafficking and health risks? Within the sociology of crime and deviance, the notion of deviance-amplification was significantly advanced by the theoretical approach known either as 'labelling theory' or 'social reaction theory' (Lemert 1951, 1967; Becker 1963). In his *Droit de la Drogue* Caballero (1989) gives eloquent expression to the many discontents which have come to surround the 'war on drugs' metaphor, while also indicating the complexities involved at attempting to arrive at a rational strategy of drug regulation.

One consequence of twentieth century history is that in spite of all that has been said about cultural diversity, drug regulation has become frozen within an increasingly centralized system of international treaties and agreements. The room for flexibility even at the margins is thereby much reduced. Moreover, within the overall framework of international regulation those societies which have experimented with different forms of 'de-criminalization' invite new problems of 'drugs tourism' — evidenced by the recent bitter conflicts in the Netherlands where border towns such as Arnhem have experienced considerable difficulties with drug users from Western Germany which has a more tightly regulated prohibitionist policy (Ephimenco 1989). Similar worries are expressed in the report of the Swiss Federal Commission (1989) which, while recommending a de-penalization of drug possession offences, recognizes that if such a policy were implemented unilaterally it would 'bring about drugs tourism in Switzerland with all the undesirable effects which this implies'.

Drug-free cultures?

Approaching culture as a 'whole way of life', we might also ask in what ways different cultures are more or less likely to generate drug problems. For example, can cultures be identified which are drug-resistant? In the broadest terms, the answer would appear to be a resounding 'No'. Even so, it might be that some cultures are less likely to use drugs in potentially harmful ways.

An interesting case is provided by Benedict's (1961) discussion of the Pueblo Indians in New Mexico, for whom sobriety was highly valued and intoxication abhorred. Unlike their neighbours such as the Apache, the Pueblo did not practise peyote-eating, and nor did they succumb to problems with alcohol when it was introduced by European settlers. Certain drug practices were however integrated into Pueblo culture, such as the use of jimson-weed (datura) to detect the identity of a thief, and tobacco smoke-blowing which was a common aspect of religious ritual and horticulture among indigenous American civilizations at the time of Columbus (Wilbert 1987).

The significant difference was that although the Pueblo used drugs, they were not used to produce states of mental excitement or visions. American Indians also employed fasting techniques as a means of generating self-induced visions. For the Pueblo, however, fasting was a means to attain ceremonial cleanliness. 'Nothing could be more unexpected to a Pueblo Indian', according to Benedict (1961), 'than any theory of a connection between fasting and any sort of exaltation'.

The place of drug use within Pueblo culture thus adds a further dimension to the comparative understanding of the relativism existing cross-culturally in terms of drugs and their uses. Not only do we find different cultures using different drugs, employing different drug-using techniques, and constructing different systems of custom and law to distinguish between appropriate forms of drug use as against those which are unacceptable. Different cultures may even use the same drugs, while at the same time the meaning of drug use is differently constructed, and the valued and desired effects of those drugs interpreted and experienced in different ways. It is at this last point that the role of pharmacology in the creation of drug-induced experiences sometimes seems to be placed in question.

SUBCULTURES AND PATTERNS OF DRUG MISUSE

The concept of subculture switches attention from how drug use varies cross-culturally, to a similar set of questions about different patterns of drug use among social groups within a single society. There is considerable local and regional variation in patterns of drug use, and the subcultural approach to drug misuse involves a wide variety of issues.

Subcultural preferences: injecting, sharing, race, and gender

As an example of this kind of phenomenon, there were distinct local variations in the impact of the heroin epidemic in the north of England in the mid-1980s (Pearson *et al.* 1985, 1986). While these variations reflected the way in which the availability of the drug remained scattered and uneven, local and regional diversity also indicated the ways in which emerging patterns of heroin use were deeply influenced by previously existing drug preferences and practices. In some localities, for example, it appeared that heroin use could not be assimilated within already existing drug subcultures. Moreover, even in those localities where heroin misuse assumed epidemic form, there were sharp contrasts in terms of the preferred mode of administration. Heroin had been previously almost unknown in most regions of the north of England, but there were nevertheless areas where injecting quickly became the preferred mode, in contrast with other areas such as Merseyside where 'chasing the dragon' was the dominant method of using the drug (Pearson *et al.* 1986; Parker *et al.* 1988).

A crucial factor in distinguishing between 'chasing' and injecting subcultures was whether there had been prior knowledge within local drug networks of powder drugs such as amphetamines, and whether powder drugs had been injected or 'snorted'. Where there were already established injecting drug subcultures, when heroin first became available in cheap and plentiful supply in the early 1980s, it was injected; whereas in areas previously unaccustomed to injection practices, although there was undoubtedly a large degree of experimentation with injecting heroin, 'chasing' remained the preferred practice (Parker *et al.* 1988; Pearson 1987a).

Subcultures within which technologies of smoking or inhalation are preferred are, without doubt, always vulnerable to the encroachment of injecting practices — predominantly because injection provides a more efficient means of using the drug, hence incurring lower financial costs to the user in maintaining his or her habit. In those localities where injecting drug subcultures prevail, on the other hand, these can prove to be extraordinarily resilient; reproducing themselves across generations of drug users, involving multiple phases of substance-transfer as different drugs become at first available and then scarce within the locality. We can see evidence of this in parts of the north-west of England and also in the cities of Edinburgh and Glasgow in Scotland. Here injecting drug cultures which were first established in the 1970s around barbiturates and amphetamines subsequently switched to heroin during the early 1980s, and then in the late 1980s embraced the injection of tranquillizers such as Temgesic and Temazepam when heroin became scarce in these areas (Morrison 1988). Local patterns of substance-transfer or 'drug-switching' have also been noted in North America (Feldman 1977). Nevertheless, one also encounters drug subcultures which remain substance-specific. One peculiar instance of this phenomenon, again found in a few towns in the north-west of England, involves the injection of cyclizine which is an anti-emetic found in a number of travel-sickness preparations (Gilman *et al.* 1990).

Subcultural variations such as these have considerable implications for the planning and effective implementation of health education programmes, treatment and rehabilitation services, and harm-reduction interventions. Another way of phrasing such variations is to say that they are a consequence of the friendship networks which assist in the acceleration of drug epidemics, but which might also contribute to their containment (Hughes and Crawford 1972; Hughes 1977). Friendship is the dominant means by which people are first introduced to drugs, so that it is once again central to effective primary prevention health education strategies (Pearson 1987a).

Attempts to reduce high-risk behaviour such as sharing injecting equipment must also contend with subcultural variations and friendship networks. The likelihood that injecting drug users will share 'works' is governed not only by the general availability of sterile injecting equipment in a locality, but also by the fact that sharing practices can be an important means by which drug users express solidarity and friendship (McKeganey 1989). North American research is also beginning to identify variations in high-risk practices between different ethnic groups such as whites, blacks, and Latinos (Wiebel 1988).

Questions of 'race' and ethnicity offer a further line of enquiry for subcultural exploration. In a multi-racial society such as contemporary Britain, a somewhat obvious question is why people of African-Caribbean origin and descent were massively under-represented within the heroin epidemic of the 1980s (Pearson 1987a). Some form of cultural opposition to heroin use is commonly assumed to have been involved, although this remains an unchallenged assumption which is difficult to square with the radically different picture in North American cities where heroin misuse has been a serious difficulty in black ghetto communities for many decades (Chein et al. 1964; Courtwright et al. 1989). There has been little attention, however, to questions of 'race' and ethnicity in research on drug use in Britain (Gabe 1988; Awiah et al. 1990; Mirza et al. 1991).

Variations in known levels of drug misuse among men and women provide another broadly based subcultural difference, but gender issues have also often been neglected in research on drug misuse (Rosenbaum 1981; Ettorre 1989). Nevertheless, gender raises important questions. Differential socialization into cultures of masculinity and femininity might, for example, imply that men are more prone to risk-taking and hence to overall higher levels of experimentation with drugs. Patriarchal assumptions within the dominant culture which define female drug users as more stigmatized, 'damaged' and 'polluted' than male drug users might even further deter women from drug experimentation, or from seeking help when women do experience drug problems. Although women are under-represented among known drug using populations, there is a gender-specific tendency for women to be much more likely to abuse other substances such as food, and the socialization of women into cultures of dependency and passivity might determine their more prevalent use of sedatives and tranquillizers (Ettorre 1986; Lawrence 1984, 1987). Graham's (1976, 1987) persuasive research on women and tobacco smoking, including smoking during pregnancy, has many implications for the future direction of gender-sensitive health education strategies.

Drug misuse and cultures of unemployment

Considerable attention has been paid to the ways in which drug subcultures are often densely concentrated within socio-economically deprived communities. In North America this has been an observable trend for many years (Chein et al. 1964; Preble and Casey 1969; Hughes 1977; Johnson et al. 1985; Williams 1989). It is a body of work which needs to be read alongside the earlier North American sociological tradition of research into delinquent subcultures (A. K. Cohen 1955; Cloward and Ohlin, 1960).

In Britain there is also a robust tradition, in the post-war years, of social research into 'youth cultures', together with delinquent and near-delinquent subcultures (Downes 1966; S. Cohen 1972; Parker 1974; Mungham and Pearson 1976; Hall and Jefferson 1976; Willis 1980; Pearson 1983). However, with a few exceptions, questions of drug misuse remain undeveloped within British research on the sociology of deviance (Young 1971a and 1971b). This neglect is in part due to the fact that criminological approaches to drug misuse are considerably undeveloped in Britain itself, reflecting the fact that the drugs–crime connection was not nearly so well established as in North America (Pearson 1990, 1991). It was not until the heroin epidemic of the 1980s, which was associated with the sharp increase in unemployment in Britain in the early 1980s, that we found confirmation of the links between drug misuse, delinquent subcultures, and social deprivation (Burr 1987; Peck and Plant 1986; Pearson 1987b; Parker et al. 1988).

The relationships between drug misuse and social deprivation work at a number of inter-connecting levels. Although the 'culture of poverty' thesis has been largely discredited, one can nevertheless point to a cultural predisposition towards risk-taking and excitement, particularly among young men who demonstrate status and achievement within poor neighbourhoods by these means (Feldman 1968). Delinquent lifestyles, involving theft and the handling of stolen goods are also available options in socio-economically deprived localities, together with other aspects of the 'informal economy' (Auld et al. 1986). It is nevertheless possible to over-state the relationships between drug-related and criminal lifestyles, as indicated by the Heroin Lifestyle Study conducted among black men in the ghettos of Chicago, New York, Washington, and Philadelphia, which demonstrated that a surprising proportion of daily heroin users were engaged in conventional forms of employment and more-or-less conventional lifestyles (Hanson et al. 1985).

We must also incorporate within this understanding of drug subcultures in poor neighbourhoods what is known about the social psychology of unemployment. One of Zinberg's (1984) significant findings is that controlled intoxicant use is more likely where a person has other valued life commitments, such as employment, which are incompatible with daily heroin use. One vitally important aspect of unemployment is the devastating impact which it makes upon an individual's routine time-structures (Jahoda et al. 1972; Jahoda, 1982). Unemployment emerges from Jahoda's research as an experience involving a profound disorientation of daily routines and time-structures (Pearson 1989). The compulsive logic of the heroin lifestyle — get straight, hustle for money, score drugs, get straight and hustle for more money — thus effectively 'solves' a major psychological burden of unemployed status (Preble and Casey 1969; Pearson 1987b).

The practical implications of the form of understanding that is beginning to be sketched out are considerable. Effective interventions in the lives of drug users must focus not only on pharmacological dependency, but must also get to grips with the active lifestyles of drug users (Gilman and Pearson 1991). One important consideration is to assist drug users in fashioning alternative modes of economic viability, while also helping them to re-structure their time routines. There is good reason to believe that when heroin users say that 'coming off' is not too much of a problem, but that 'staying off' is exceptionally difficult, a major part of this difficulty is how to re-structure one's lifestyle which had become a major source of identity, meaning, and time management.

Cultures of employment: musicians, medics, and prostitutes

One aspect of a society which relies upon an extensive division of labour is that it is characterized by a variety of occupational and professional subcultures. How do these interact with patterns of drug use? The lifestyle associated with a valued employment status is under most circumstances incompatible with a drug practice such as daily heroin use. There are, however, a small number of cases where it is not incompatible and which have particular interest for any consideration of the cultural contexts of drug misuse. These tend to be occupations of an expressive or creative nature, and principally in the music industry. Some aspects of this terrain are explored in Howard Becker's essay on dance band musicians, and we obtain glimpses of what is involved in biographies such as that of jazz saxophonist Charlie Parker (Becker 1955; Russell 1973; Courtwright et al. 1989; Shapiro 1988).

As with other subcultural forms of drug use, a number of factors appear to be at work. Certain forms of drug use can be experienced as aids to creativity. In appropriate doses cannabis would not appear to interrupt the psycho-motor functions necessary for effective musicianship of the jazz/rock variety, and might assist in the process of 'improvisation'. It has also been suggested that the development of American jazz from 'hot' to 'cool' — from Dixieland, to swing, to modern jazz 'bop' — was associated with changing drug preferences among jazz musicians from alcohol, to marijuana, and then to heroin (Winick 1959, 1961).

Within the occupational cultures of musicianship, drug use also signifies 'hipness' — that is, identification with the bohemian subculture which surrounds the jazz or rock scene, and distance from (or rejection of) the 'straight' world of nine-to-five conformity. Even so, it is only controlled drug use which is compatible with successful musicianship (Winick 1961). Where drug use slips out of control, as in the numerous personal and professional tragedies which litter the path of popular and avant-garde music, the musician's art is eventually destroyed — sometimes along with the musician. Nevertheless, he or she is not then rejected by the culture of jazz music as a 'drop-out' or 'failure' — which would be the case if a successful businessman or academic succumbed to an addiction. Rather, they become exemplars of the culture and its internal contradictions. The heroes and heroines in the tragic mode of the jazz/rock music world thus define the limits of a culture. It is in this sense that drug use and drug casualties can be said to be fully integrated within its occupational culture — which is not to minimize the resulting individual tragedies.

There are no doubt other employment statuses where drug use is either not incompatible with successful accomplishment, or deemed even necessary for it — coca chewing by miners in the Andes; stimulant use by soldiers under certain combat conditions; the 'business lunch'. The use of ganja among some people in the Caribbean as an aid to hard physical labour provides a further example, while also illustrating the way in which cultural contexts can radically alter the meanings and experiences associated with the use of a drug (Rubin and Comitas 1975). It seems unlikely, however, that there are other occupational cultures comparable to music where drug use is so fully integrated that self-destruction assumes the form of heroism.

The place of drug misuse within medicine involves a number of factors (Winick 1964, 1974; Hessler 1974). There is an easier availability to dangerous drugs, which is always a necessary condition for drug use. Medical practitioners are also more familiar with methods of drug administration such as intravenous injection, and therefore less constrained by cultural taboos against self-injection. Finally, there is the role which the medical profession unwittingly plays in the dissemination of the dominant cultural attitude that a pill is a cure for a variety of complaints. Given the role of medicine within this general cultural framework, it seems likely that the occupational culture of medicine will embody this attitude in an intensified form.

Prostitution is another occupational subculture which is associated with systematic drug use, and where closer attention to gender questions is again required in our understanding of problem drug use (Plant 1990). The connection between prostitution and heroin misuse has often been remarked upon (Rosenbaum 1981; Courtwright *et al.* 1989). The 'crack' problem in the USA also appears to have become deeply associated with prostitution (Bourgois 1989). Recent research in the Netherlands indicates that there are a number of different routes by which the heroin–prostitute phenomenon occurs, and that this is not only associated with different subcultural meanings of both heroin use and prostitution, but that it also has implications for treatment and rehabilitation strategies (Blom and van den Berg 1989).

CULTURE AS THE 'CULTIVATION OF HABITS': SOCIALIZATION, PHARMACOLOGY, AND CULTURE

Already at a number of points in the earlier discussion — concerning the Pueblos, for example, or ganja use as an aid to agricultural labour in the Caribbean — the perspective of cultural relativism had begun to shade into a related but different set of questions. These concern the social meanings which surround drugs and drug use in any given culture or subculture, and how the question of drug use is socially constructed. There are three overlapping issues to be addressed here which it is not always possible to disentangle.

The first is the question of whether and how the cultural meanings which are attached to drugs influence the attitudes, belief systems, and lifestyles of drug users. The second concerns whether and how the cultural meanings which are attached to drugs influence the experience of drug use, in the sense of the perceived and desired psychopharmacological effects of drugs. The third focuses on the ways in which drug users are socialized into the specific sets of meanings and beliefs of any given drug subculture.

The Becker thesis: becoming a marijuana user

In his seminal essays on 'Becoming a marijuana user' and 'Marijuana use and social control', Howard Becker promoted an argument that the process of becoming a marijuana user is essentially a learning experience (Becker 1953a, b). This learning takes place through interaction with more experienced users, and it is through these interactions rather than through the direct and unmediated pharmacological effects of the drug that the novice user learns how to be a successful marijuana user — that is, how to 'get high'. Indeed, a starting point for Becker and for many other commentators was that 'the novice does not ordinarily get high the first time he smokes marijuana, and several attempts are usually necessary to induce this state'.

First, Becker suggested, the novice user had to learn the technique of smoking the drug, inhaling a sufficient quantity of the fumes, etc. The next step was 'learning to perceive the effects'. Finally, the novice had to 'learn to enjoy the effects' since these might initially be experienced as ambiguous, unpleasant, or even frightening. Only when the novice user has learned to re-interpret these sensations as enjoyable is he or she 'willing and able to use marijuana for pleasure'.

A number of points need to be made about Becker's approach. The first is that although it has often been understood as having specific reference only to cannabis use, it is undoubtedly an approach to drug experimentation with a more general application. The dizziness caused by the first cigarette or the first intake of alcohol in any quantity, or the experience of nausea initially experienced by heroin users — these are all ambiguous and potentially unpleasant drug effects which need to be re-interpreted within a cultural framework of pleasure-seeking (Pearson et al. 1986; Pearson 1987a).

Becker's account nevertheless seriously risks underestimating the role of pharmacology, and has certainly given encouragement to those who promote the idea that cannabis is 'pharmacologically little more than a placebo' (Auld 1973). Research which aimed to test Becker's scheme of initiation into drug experiences among a group of cannabis users encountered a variety of forms of disbelief about the necessity of 'learning to experience the effects', neatly summed up in the remark that 'that guy Becker should change his dealer!' (Pearson and Twohig 1975). Closer attention needs to be given to the technologies of smoking cannabis — whether it is smoked in tobacco-rolled joints, for example, or whether it is used without tobacco; whether the drug is initially tried after consuming alcohol, and so on — factors which might imply different learning experiences, and possibly different psychopharmacologies.

The more general question is the role afforded to pharmacology in interpretive schemes such as Becker's. The mediating role of culture — in the form of shared meanings, activities, and symbolism — seems to be undeniable. The emphasis on cultural 'set and setting', which was further extended in Becker's (1967) essay on LSD psychosis, also seems entirely justifiable on the basis of a range of sociological and anthropological research. However, this is not to say that pharmacology can be eliminated from our understanding of drug use. Indeed, to do so would be to succumb to a vulgar form of philosophical idealism. How do we, then, formulate the relationships between the constancies of pharmacology and the variations at an experiental level, in the differences to which the same drug can be put, and the different drug-induced experiences which can result from the same drug?

Pharmacology and culture: The 'raw' and the 'cooked'

If we are to remain faithful to a materialist philosophy of science, then due acknowledgement must be given to the place of pharmacology within drug experiences — even though those experiences might be subject to widespread modification through a variety of cultural influences. The question of drug use is not in any sense unique in this respect. Fundamental areas of human experience and human self-understanding involve a collision between a universally agreed biology and a range of cultural meanings which are attached to it — whether we think of rituals associated with biological mechanisms such as menstruation, historical and cross-cultural variations transcribed upon human sexuality, or the diversity of cuisines and 'tastes' which divide and separate the essential bodily requirements of nutrition (Douglas 1978; Ortner and Whitehead 1981; Levi-Strauss 1978).

This issue can be further elaborated by references to Paul Willis's (1978) *Profane Culture*, which offers an ethnographic study of two distinct subcultures of motor-bike boys and hippies. In several respects, he advances a similar argument to Becker's. In his discussion of drug use among hippies, which was largely confined to cannabis and LSD, he suggests that 'drugs were only inverted placebos, keys to experience, rather than experience'. Nevertheless, he does concede a place to pharmacology. Within the hippie subculture, high status was afforded to those people known as 'heads', and Willis suggests that they were also more likely to employ higher dosage levels than casual smokers of cannabis:

The serious head smoker inhaled very much more deeply, and kept the smoke in the lungs very much longer, than did the casual user. He was also very much more likely to control the amount of the drug, during the ritualistic making of the 'joint', at a high consistent level than was the casual smoker ... The ritualistic practices, then, which grew to surround the drug both increased the 'raw' effect they had on consciousness (through greater ingestion) and resonated this experience in a particular way (through greater focusing of the circumstances of ingestion). The greater raw experience thus provided gave more scope for appropriate cultural interpretation, which in turn facilitated more intensive smoking rituals, producing higher levels of ingestion, etc., etc.

In this way, Willis developed a careful account of a dialectical process between pharmacology (the 'raw' effect) and ritual, which attempts to remain faithful to the hippie 'head' phenomenon. There is a continuing assumption that it is the ambiguous nature of the 'raw' effect produced by hallucinogens which allows space for varied systems of interpretation. Adopting a stance similar to the concept of drug 'plasticity' introduced by Edwards (1974), this is set against the possibility that the 'raw' effects set limits to the scope for the cultural interpretation of drug experiences.

When Willis turns to heroin use, which was much less common within the hippie subculture which he studied, his account of 'the particular chemical effects of different drugs and their interaction with cultural meanings' shifts its emphasis. Heroin 'had, as it were, only a one-way relationship with the culture', rather than one in which pharmacology and culture were understood in a dialogue with each other:

It was an unanswerable closure... clear evidence that the heroin drug experience could not be influenced and moulded as could that of acid or hash... In this sense we see a very clear limitation of cultural meaning set by the pharmacological basis of a drug' (Willis 1978).

CASE STUDIES: LSD AND HEROIN

Working within broadly the same conceptual framework as Becker, Willis's approach is a significant development on Becker's more rudimentary scheme, in that it offers a much more explicit and elaborated account of the interplay of pharmacology and culture. We must nevertheless enter some final questions which will be approached by means of two case studies on the subcultural interpretations of LSD and heroin. The first of these case studies will examine the status of the concept of 'set and setting' which has been so influential in shaping debates on the cultural contexts of drug use. The second approaches the interaction of pharmacology, culture, and language through an examination of the varied accounts which heroin users give of their experiences with the drug.

'Set and setting': the sixties' influence

In its barest essentials, the 'set and setting' approach takes the view that the perceived effects of a drug will be decisively altered by the mood and attitude set of the person at the time the drug is ingested, and further influenced by the physical and social setting within which drug use occurs (Zinberg 1984). My argument will be that although the concept of 'set and setting' has enjoyed a privileged status within these debates, it is also one that is flawed. In a large measure, the concept drew its legitimacy from the drug subculture of the 1960s, and both its strengths and its difficulties derive from this. What has been commonly ignored in discussions on 'set and setting' is the contradictory nature of the belief system of the 1960s drug culture, involving a deep fracture-line on the role of pharmacology in LSD experiences.

As we have seen, the view that culture could have a significant influence on the subjective experience of drug use, and that this might also be decisive in determining the outcome of an individual's or group's experimentation with a variety of drugs, was already available prior to the 1960s, both through anthropological evidence and also through the influential contributions of Lindesmith (1947) and Becker (1953a, b). It was, however, a view which was to be dramatically reinforced by the drug cultures of the 1960s — specifically those middle class drug cultures associated with hallucinogens and 'psychedelics', notably cannabis and LSD.

As revealed by Jay Stevens' (1989) social history of LSD in America, *Storming Heaven*, prior to its emergence as a dominant influence within the 1960s drug culture, a number of quite distinct interest groups had already converged on LSD: laboratory scientists exploring the chemical correlates of psychotic illnesses, for whom the drug was a psychotomimetic; psychotherapists, for whom it promised an express-way to the unconscious; the CIA for whom it was a potential agent in chemical warfare; avant-garde artists for whom it promised intensified levels of creativity; a variety of mystics and intellectuals, such as Aldous Huxley, for whom it promised enhanced human powers; and an assortment of crackpots and dreamers. In other words, LSD was already wrapped up within a number of utterly distinct and separate cultures, and its social meaning differed within each of these social groups. LSD offers a case-study, in fact, of how the same chemical substance can be appropriated within a variety of different cultures of meaning.

The 1960s drug culture was to appropriate the drug within another constellation of meanings, most closely related to those of the psychotherapists, avant-garde artists, mystics, and intellectuals. It is generally accepted that the 'hippie' exploration of 'inner space' was deeply influenced by Huxley and Leary who placed a central emphasis on the importance of 'set and setting' in determining the outcomes of an LSD experience — advocating the use of the drug in a framework of quiet contemplation.

The centrality of 'set and setting' was further reinforced by the question of the 'bad trip' which, as experience was gained with LSD within the emerging drug culture, was to become part of the folk culture of the hippie movement centred on Haight Ashbury. Becker again made a significant impact on the tone and structure of the debate with his paper of 1967 on 'History, culture and subjective experience' which reviewed what was known about the question of 'LSD psychosis'. A further contribution to this debate was the paper by Munoz and Davis (1968) on 'Heads and freaks' which examined 'patterns and meanings of drug use among hippies' in the aftermath of the 'Summer of Love' in Haight Ashbury.

If we follow Munoz and Davis, the fragmentation which emerged within the 1960s drug culture assumed a specific form between the cool 'heads' and hedonistic 'freaks'. In part, this came from the diversification of hippie drug practices to include not only cannabis and LSD but also methedrine. The use of 'speed' had been already known for some years within California motor cycle gangs such as Hell's Angels. Its acceptance within some segments of the hippie community also led to an altered approach to drug use: for kicks rather than self exploration and meditation.

This split between 'heads' and 'freaks' also resulted from a tension within the 'psychedelic' movement itself, which has often gone unrecognized in discussions on 'set and setting'. Although Leary and others adopted the philosophy of set and setting, which was followed by the 'heads' and those who had become interested in Eastern religions and other 'far-out' belief systems, on the West Coast 'acid scene' the pace was set by Ken Kesey and his Pranksters, aptly characterized by Tom Wolfe's (1969) *Electric Kool-Aid Acid Test* as a madhouse of the wild, unruly, libidinal approach to the liberation of a generation.

There was therefore no general agreement on the 'set and setting' argument from within the drug culture itself. Indeed, there was no such thing as a unified and homogeneous drug culture. The 'heads' employed the philosophy of set and setting in order to achieve self-insight and to enhance 'mind-expanding' experiences. The 'freaks' embraced a hedonistic attitude whereby LSD was associated with 'tripping' in the context of light-shows and rock bands. There was little love lost between these two groups. As described by Munoz and Davis (1968), those 'who used LSD only to "trip"' were 'regarded at best, with a certain amused tolerance by "righteous acid heads"'.

One final aspect of this fragmentation within the 'psychedelic' culture, also noted by Munoz and Davis, directly challenged the view that the role of pharmacology should be subordinated to other considerations. If one side of the drug culture emphasized the crucial centrality of 'set and setting' in determining the outcome of LSD sessions, there was a competing tendency within the psychedelic movement which placed an emphasis on the psychopharmacology of the drug itself — as something which 'opened the door' to altered states of consciousness and contemplation. Allen Ginsberg's response to his first LSD experience was phrased in this way: 'This drug seems to automatically produce a mystical experience. Science is getting very hip' (Miles 1989).

It is important to stress that this was held as a position within the drug-using subculture itself — rather than something imposed from outside by social scientists. Moreover, to argue for the truth or falsity of these two competing belief-systems is perhaps to miss the point. The more significant issue is that they indicate a contradiction within what is more commonly approached as a unified and coherent philosophy of 'set and setting' as the necessary prerequisite for the desired state of consciousness. The belief-system of 'set and setting' was no more than one specific set of cultural meanings which attached themselves to the LSD experience, counterposed by the equally authentic belief-system which stressed the primacy of pharmacology.

Heroin and experience: the limits of language

No-one would suggest that heroin is a 'placebo'. Rather, it is understood as a pharmacologically powerful agent. Nevertheless, the accounts of heroin users are plagued by ambiguity in their responses to the drug — even when one discounts those people who found that opiates initially produced unpleasant feelings of nausea (Pearson *et al.* 1986; Pearson 1987a). Here, by way of illustration, are a few examples of heroin users talking about their initial experiences.

Not uncommonly, heroin users find it difficult to convey in a precise manner the effects of the the drug, so that the description is set in a characteristic vagueness:

First, when I was on it, like, I donnow ... it made me feel dead pleasant, I donnow, dead ... as if I never had a care in the world, d'you know what I mean? It wasn't like a 'high' ... You know exactly what you're doing and all that. It was just, like ... you haven't got a care, y'know, it was just different
(Paul, 24 years, Merseyside)

For others, heroin's effects are described in straightforward and immediate terms, as simply pleasureable:

It's just the nicest drug going, you feel just great! Just ... phoo ... blows our mind, like, you start nodding and ...
(Eddie, 21 years, Merseyside)

What, however, is the precise nature of this pleasurable experience? Where does it stand along a spectrum from peaceful relaxation to intense excitement? For some, heroin's effects were slow and relaxing:

With smoking, it comes on you gradually ... and you just feel dead relaxed and dead tired and what have you ...
(Mick, 23 years, Manchester)

For others, its effects were immediate and urgent, associated with a feeling of great personal strength and power:

As soon as you chase it, it just hits you straight away ... and you just feel like the boss, like ...
(Jack, 22 years, Merseyside)

It was just ... whoosh ... an instant hit, you know, like the best high ever ...'
(Barry, 22 years, Manchester)

Whereas another form of response might appeal to the feeling of being 'wrecked' and helpless:

And the hit's brilliant, when you first start. Like, you sit there ... and it's just like, helpless. You must look bad and all that, cos I've seen my mates and thought they did ... But like, I'm just sitting there gouching ... it's brilliant
(John, 19 years, Merseyside)

Finally, there are those heroin users who give an uncomplicated response within the terms of the available vocabulary of the drug culture:

I liked the buzz I got'
(Wendy, 21 years, South Yorkshire)

These accounts indicate a remarkable diversity in the responses to heroin's effects. In attempting to explain this diversity, the first thing to note is that these responses are not drawn from an exotic cross-cultural perspective, such as that revealed by social anthropology. They thus offer a powerful statement in support of the plasticity of pharmacology.

These variations might perhaps in part reflect the experiences of different individuals with different drugs prior to their initial involvement with heroin. Someone who had previously been accustomed to amphetamines would no doubt be impressed with the soothing properties of opiates, thus influencing their perception and interpretation of heroin's effects.

The more general question, however, concerns the role of language and how one gives voice to internal states of experience, such as those induced by mind-altering drugs. Contemporary drug cultures make available only a very limited vocabulary with which to describe such internal states. This stands in sharp contrast to the dictionaries which can be compiled to identify drugs themselves. Even when one listens to those who are adepts within the drugs scene, there is a paucity within the culture with regard to words which describe drug effects. The vocabulary such as it is — 'buzz', 'stoned', 'wrecked', 'spaced out', 'high' — is not one which describes very much, although this already comes close to exhausting this narrow lexicon. Moreover, these same words are commonly employed by drug users in order to describe the effects of quite different pharmacological agents — cannabis, heroin, amphetamines, cocaine.

One means by which we can distinguish different cultures and their material practices, is the extent to which their associated languages offer sharply differentiated attention to the required functions of language. For example, the Nuer people of the Sudan whose traditional culture focuses around a dominant preoccupation with cattle, had evolved 'a vast vocabulary relating to them and their needs' (Evans-Pritchard 1956) including an elaborate system of terms to distinguish cattle by their physical markings. Similarly, a defining quality of specialized subcultures (whether these are occupational subcultures or deviant subcultures) is that they devise their own specialized vocabularies — slang or argot. For whatever reason, it would appear that internal states of experience have not assumed a high priority in the evolution of specialist vocabularies within drug-using subcultures.

This might seem to imply that the paucity of linguistic improvisation within drug cultures reflects the paucity of these cultures themselves. However, there is another way of approaching the matter. One function of culture is to simplify, and render available in a mutually agreeable and comprehensible form, the multiplicities of human experience. Culture re-orders a complex world as something which can be 'taken-for-granted'. It offers recipes for action which might otherwise be bogged down into indecision. Alfred Schutz (1964) puts the matter this way:

Thus it is the function of the cultural pattern to eliminate troublesome inquiries by offering ready-made directions for use, to replace truth hard to attain by comfortable truisms, and to substitute the self-explanatory for the questionable.

One of the central aspects of shared experience within a drug culture is, of course, the use of drugs. A major preoccupation within the culture thereby becomes how to communicate descriptions and accounts of internal states, which by their very nature are 'private' and 'unknowable' to others, in a form that is available to others in a comprehensible way. Hence, we might say that a central function of the specialized vocabulary of a drug culture will be to narrow down the ample scope for confusion in communicating the essentially incommunicable.

Different cultures order their vocabularies of meaning and motivation in different ways, for a variety of human activities. The 'inedible' raw material of human experience is thus rendered amenable within the cultural pressure-cooker which transforms it into a recognizable shared entity. The indecision about how to identify and label internal states of experience which is evident in the accounts of drug users, until they affiliate to a focused network of other users among whom a vocabulary of experience and motivation is agreed and ratified, is perhaps necessarily diffuse.

The study of true placebo effects tells us that individuals respond differently, sometimes according to questions of personality and temperament, to imagined bodily invasions. There should then be no oddity in the fact that individual human beings respond and react differently to the subjective realm, where real pharmacological agents are concerned. On the one hand, where such differences occur, they may be ironed out and concealed within the linguistic recipes supplied by specific cultures. On the other, if one were to assume that the 'raw' experience of drugs is the same for all human subjects, the linguistic devices available in different cultures and subcultures might render this experience differently in speech acts.

Our study of the cultural contexts of drug experiences may, thus, be limited precisely by the nature of culture itself — that is, by the constraints placed upon us by the limiting functions of available and improvised languages which serve to communicate the solipsism of drug experience.

REFERENCES

Auld, J. (1973). Cannabis: the changing patterns of Use. *New Society*, 6th September 1973.

Auld, J., Dorn, N., and South, N. (1986). Irregular work, irregular pleasures: heroin in the 1980s. In Matthews, R. and Young, J. (eds) *Confronting crime*. Sage, London.

Awiah, J., Butt, S., and Dorn, N. (1990). 'The last place I would go': black people and drug services in Britain. *Druglink*, 5, no. 5, 14–15.

Becker, H. S. (1953a). Becoming a marijuana user. *American Journal of Sociology*, LIX, November 1953. [Reprinted in Becker, H. S., *Outsiders*, op. cit.]

Becker, H. S. (1953b). Marijuana use and social control. *Human organization*, 12, Spring 1953. [Reprinted in Becker, H. S., *Outsiders*, op. cit.]

Becker, H. S. (1955). Careers in a deviant occupational group: the dance musician. *Social Problems*, 3, [Reprinted in Becker, H. S., *Outsiders*, op. cit.]

Becker, H. S. (1963). *Outsiders: studies in the sociology of deviance*. Free Press, New York.

Becker, H.S. (1967). History, culture and subjective experience: an exploration of the social bases of drug-induced experiences. *Journal of Health and Social Behaviour*, 8, 163–76. [Reprinted in Becker, H. S. (1971)]. *Sociological work*. Allen Lane, London.

Benedict, R. (1961). *Patterns of culture*. Routledge & Kegan Paul, London.

Berridge, V. and Edwards, G. (1981). *Opium and the people: opiate use in nineteenth century England*. Allen Lane, London. (2nd edn Yale University Press, New Haven 1987).

M. Blom and T. Van Den Berg (1989). A typology of the life and work of 'heroin-prostitutes'. In Cain, M. (ed.), *Growing up good: policing the behaviour of girls in Europe*. Sage, London.

Bourgois, P. (1989). Crack in Spanish Harlem: culture and economy in the inner city. *Anthropology Today*, 5, no. 4, pp. 6–11.

Burr, A. (1987). Chasing the dragon: heroin misuse, delinquency and crime in the context of South London Culture, *British Journal of Criminology*, 27, no. 4, 333–57.

Caballero, F. (1989). *Droit de la drogue*. Dalloz, Paris.

Carstairs, G. M. (1954). Bhang and alcohol: cultural factors in the choice of intoxicants. *Quarterly Journal of Studies on Alcohol*, 15, 220–37. [Reprinted in Solomon, D. (ed.) (1969). *The marijuana papers*. Panther, London.

Chein, I., Gerard, D., Lee, R., and Rosenfeld, E. (1964). *The road to H: narcotics, delinquency and social policy*. Tavistock, London.

Cloward, R. and Ohlin, L. (1960). *Delinquency and opportunity: a theory of delinquent gangs*. Free Press, New York.

Cohen, A. K. (1955). *Delinquent boys*. Free Press, New York:
Cohen, S. (1972). *Folk devils and moral panics: the creation of the Mods and Rockers*. MacGibbon & Kee, London.
Courtwright, D., Joseph, H., and Des Jarlais D. (1989). *Addicts who survived: an oral history of narcotic use in America, 1923–1965*. University of Tennessee Press, Knoxville.
Douglas, M. (1978). *Purity and danger: an analysis of the concepts of pollution and taboo*. Routledge & Kegan Paul, London.
Downes, D. (1966). *The delinquent solution*. Routledge & Kegan Paul, London.
Edwards, G. (1974). Drug dependence and plasticity. *Quarterly Journal of Studies on Alcohol*, **35**, 176–95.
Ephimenco, S. (1989). Arnhem livre aux cróises antidrogue. *Liberation*, 27 September 1989, p. 23.
Ettorre, B. (1986). Psychotropics, passivity and the pharmaceutical industry. In Henman, A. et al. (eds) *Big deal: the politics of the illicit drug business*. Pluto, London.
Ettorre, B. (1989). Women, substance abuse and self-help. In MacGregor, S. (ed.) *Drugs and british society*. Routledge, London.
Evans-Pritchard, E. E. (1956). *Nuer religion*. Oxford University Press, Oxford.
Fay, P. W. (1976). *The Opium War 1840–1842*. Norton, New York.
Feldman, H. W. (1968). Ideological supports to becoming and remaining a heroin addict. *Journal of Health and Social Behaviour*, **9**, 131–9.
Feldman, H. W. (1977). A neighbourhood history of drug switching. In Weppner, R. S. (ed.) *Street ethnography*. Sage, London.
Gabe, J. (1988). 'Race' and tranquilliser use. In Dorn, N., Lucas, L., and South, N. (eds) *Drug questions*, Research Register issue 4. ISDD, London.
Gilman, M. and Pearson, G. (1991). Lifestyles and law enforcement. In P. Bean & Whynes, D. K. (eds) *Policing and prescribing: the British system of drug control*. Macmillan, London.
Gilman, M., Traynor, P., and Pearson, G. (1990). 'The limits of intervention: cyclizine misuse. *Druglink*, **5**, no. 3, pp. 12–13.
Graham, H. (1976). Smoking in pregnancy: the attitudes of expectant mothers. *Social Science and Medicine*, **10**, 399–405.
Graham, H. (1987). Women's smoking and family health. *Social Science and Medicine*, **25**, 47–56.
Hall, S. and Jefferson, T. (eds) (1976). *Resistance through rituals*. Hutchinson, London.
Hanson, B., Beschner, G., Walters, J. M., and Bovelle, E. (1985). *Life with heroin: voices from the Inner City*. Lexington, Lexington, Massachusetts.
Hessler, R. M. (1974). Junkies in white: drug addiction among physicians. In Bryant, C. D. (ed.) *Deviant behaviour: occupational and organisational bases*. Rand McNally, Chicago.
Hughes, P. H. (1977). *Behind the wall of respect: community experiments in heroin addiction control*. University of Chicago Press, Chicago.
Hughes, P. H. and Crawford, G. A. (1972). A contagious disease model for researching and intervening in heroin epidemics. *Archives of General Psychiatry*, **27**, 189–205.

Jahoda, M. (1982). *Employment and unemployment: a social-psychological analysis.* Cambridge University Press, Cambridge.
Jahoda, M., Lazarsfeld, P., and Zeisel, H. (1972). *Marienthal: the Sociography of an unemployed community.* Tavistock, London.
Johnson, B. D., Goldstein, P. J., Preble, E., Schmeidler, J. Lipton, D. S., Spunt, B., and Miller, T. (1985). *Taking care of business: the economics of crime by heroin abusers.* Lexington, Lexington, Massachusetts.
Lawrence, M. (1984). *The anorexic experience.* Women's Press, London.
Lawrence, M. (ed.) (1987). *Fed up and hungry: women, oppression and food.* Women's Press, London.
Lemert, E. M. (1951). *Social pathology.* McGraw–Hill, New York.
Lemert, E. M. (1967). *Human deviance, social problems and social control.* Prentice–Hall, New Jersey.
Lévi-Strauss, C. (1978). *The origin of table manners: introduction to a science of mythology,* Vol. 3. Jonathan Cape, London.
Lindesmith, A. R. (1947). *Opiate addiction.* Principia Press, Bloomington.
McKeganey, N. (1989). Drug abuse in the community: needle-sharing and the risks of HIV infection. In Cunningham-Burley, S. and McKeganey, N. (eds) *Readings in medical sociology.* Routledge, London.
Miles, B. (1989). *Ginsberg: a biography.* Viking, London.
Mirza, H. S. Pearson, G., and Phillips, S. (1991). *Drugs, people and services in Lewisham: final report of the drug information project.* University of London, Goldsmiths' College, London.
Morrison, V. (1988). Drug misuse and concern about HIV infection in Edinburgh: an interim report. In Dorn, N. Lucas, L. and South, N. (eds), *Drug questions,* Research Register issue 4. ISDD, London.
Mungham, G. and Pearson, G. (eds) (1976). *Working class youth culture.* Routledge & Kegan Paul, London.
Munoz, L. and Davis, F. (1968). Heads and freaks: patterns and meanings of drug use among hippies. *Journal of Health and Social Behaviour,* **9**, 156–64.
Musto, D. (1973). *The American disease: origins of narcotic control.* Yale University Press, New Haven.
Ortner, S. B. and H. Whitehead (eds) (1981). *Sexual meanings: the cultural construction of gender and sexuality.* Cambridge University Press, Cambridge.
Parker, H. (1974). *View from the boys.* David & Charles, London.
Parker, H., Bakx, K., and Newcombe, R. (1988). *Living with heroin: the impact of a drugs epidemic on an English Community.* Open University Press, Milton Keynes.
Pearson, G. (1983). *Hooligan: a history of respectable fears.* Macmillan, London.
Pearson, G. (1985). Lawlessness, modernity and social change: a historical appraisal. *Theory, culture and society,* **2**, no. 3, 15–35.
Pearson, G. (1987*a*). *The new heroin users.* Blackwell, Oxford.
Pearson, G. (1987*b*). 'Social deprivation, unemployment and patterns of heroin use. In Dorn, N. and South, N. (eds) *A land fit for heroin? Drug policies, prevention and practice.* Macmillan, London.
Pearson, G. (1989). Women and men without work: the political economy is personal. In Rojek, C. et al. (eds), *The haunt of misery: critical essays in social work and helping.* Routledge, London.

Pearson, G. (1990). Drugs, law enforcement and criminology. In Berridge, V. (ed.) *Drugs research and policy in Britain*. Avebury, Aldershot.
Pearson, G. (1991). British drug control policy. In Tonry, M. and Morris, N. (eds) *Crime and justice*, Vol. 14. University of Chicago Press.
Pearson, G. and Twohig, J. (1975). Ethnography through the looking-glass: the case of Howard Becker. *Working Papers in Cultural Studies*, no. 7/8, 1975, 119-25. [Reprinted in Hall, S. and Jefferson, T. (eds) (1976). *Resistance through rituals*. Hutchinson, London.]
Pearson, G., Gilman, M., and McIver, S. (1985). Heroin use in the north of England. *Health Education Journal*, 45, no. 3, pp. 186-9.
Pearson, G., Gilman, M., and McIver, S. (1986). *Young people and heroin: an examination of heroin use in the north of England*. Health Education Council, London and Gower, Aldershot.
Peck, D. F. and Plant, M.A. (1986). Unemployment and illegal drug use: concordant evidence from a prospective study and national trends. *British Medical Journal*, 239, 929-32.
Plant, M. A. (ed.) (1990) *AIDS, drugs and prostitution*. Routledge, London.
Preble, E. and Casey, J.J. (1969). Taking care of business: the heroin user's life on the street. *International Journal of Addictions*, 4, no. 1, 1-24.
Rosenbaum, M. (1981). *Women on heroin*. Rutgers University Press, New Brunswick, New Jersey.
Rubin, V. and Comitas, L. (1975). *Ganja in Jamaica: a medical anthropological study of chronic marihuana use*. Mouton, The Hague.
Russell, R. (1973). *Bird lives! The high life and hard times of Charlie 'Yardbird' Parker*. Quartet, London.
Schutz, A. (1964). The stranger: an essay in social psychology. In Schutz, A., *Collected papers II: studies in social theory*. Martinus Nijhoff, The Hague.
Shapiro, H. (1988). *Waiting for the man: the story of drugs and popular music*. Quartet, London.
Stevens, J. (1989). *Storming heaven: LSD and the American dream*. Paladin, London.
Swiss Federal Commission (1989). *Aspects de la Situation et de la politique en matière de drogue en Suisse*. Office Fédéral de la Santé Publique, Berne.
Tylor, E. B. (1871). *Primitive culture: researches into the development of mythology, philosophy, religion, language, art, and custom*. 2 Vols. John Murray, London.
Wiebel, W. W. (1988). Combining ethnographic and epidemiological methods in targetted AIDS interventions: the Chicago model. In Battjes, R.J. and Pickens, R. W. (eds) *Needle sharing among intravenous drug abusers: national and international perspectives*, NIDA Research Monograph 80. NIDA, Rockville, Maryland.
Wilbert, J. (1987). *Tobacco and shamanism in South America*. Yale University Press, New Haven.
Williams, R. (1983). *Keywords*. Flamingo, London.
Williams, T. (1989). *The cocaine kids*. Addison-Wesley, New York.
Willis, P. (1978). *Profane culture*. Routledge & Kegan Paul, London.
Willis, P. (1980). *Learning to labour*. Gower, Aldershot.

Winick, C. (1959). The use of drugs by jazz musicians. *Social Problems*, 7, 240–53.
Winick, C. (1961). How high the moon: jazz and drugs. *Antioch review*, Spring 1961, 53–68.
Winick, C. (1964). Physician narcotic addicts. In Becker, H. S. (ed.) *The other side: perspectives on deviance*. Free Press, New York.
Winick, C. (1974). Drug dependence among nurses. In Winick, C. (ed.) *Sociological aspects of drug dependence*. CRC Press, Cleveland, Ohio.
Wolfe, T. (1969). *The electric kool-aid acid test*. Bantam, New York.
Young, J. (1971*a*). The role of the police as amplifiers of deviance, negotiators of reality and translators of fantasy. In Cohen, S. (ed.) *Images of deviance*. Penguin, Harmondsworth.
Young, J. (1971*b*). *The drugtakers*. Paladin, London.
Zinberg, N. E. (1984). *Drug, set, and setting: the basis for controlled intoxicant use*. Yale University Press, New Haven.

8

Detecting individual factors in substance abuse problems

LEE ROBINS

There has been a long standing argument in the substance abuse field, over whether use at a level that creates problems should or should not be considered a psychiatric disorder. One of the arguments against the psychiatric view is that the level of substance use determines whether there will be problems, and level of use is largely culturally determined — either as specified by the main culture or a subculture to which the individual belongs, or by the degree of stress that the culture creates for the individual — rather than being a sign of a malfunctioning *individual*.

To move this old argument at least one step toward resolution, we need to consider how one would go about deciding whether substance abuse problems are of cultural or individual origin. We will consider as 'individual' factors those in which there is an enduring vulnerability in the individual, even if that vulnerability may have its roots in an earlier cultural experience. We believe this is the ordinary understanding. For example, death by shooting has an 'unnatural' cause because the injury is typically brief prior to the death. Death by cancer has a 'natural' cause even if the cancer itself could be explained in large part by exposure to environmental toxins, because the direct cause is an enduring lesion in the individual. There are, unfortunately, difficult cases even here — for example, when the person shot survives briefly but dies a month later from an infection at the wound site. But we will dodge these difficulties as far as possible by ignoring ultimate causes, while attempting to distinguish proximal causes that are cultural from those that are individual. Although one can certainly argue that distal causes are at least as important conceptually and practically as proximal causes, they rapidly lead one into an infinite regression — not only back to one's own environment of rearing but from there to one's parents' early environment.

A STRATEGY FOR IDENTIFYING LIKELY INDIVIDUAL CONTRIBUTORS

It seems reasonable to argue that individual differences must explain the fact that members of the same cultural group can differ from each other with respect to substance abuse problems. Individual differences will determine whether the cultural guidelines with respect to use will be followed or violated, and for those following cultural guidelines, whether their use will fall near the bottom or top of the permitted range. Individual variation in biological and psychological make-up (perhaps allergies to drugs, diseased livers, poor judgement in engaging in incompatible activities while using intoxicants, or poorly controlled aggressiveness that is released by disinhibiting drugs), will cause problems for some even though they use substances at culturally prescribed levels. The more detailed the cultural prescriptions with respect to what to use, when to use it, and how to ingest it, the more uniform will use be, and therefore the clearer it will be that the variation in substance abuse problems among adherents to the rules can be attributed to individual variation.

When we undertake the task of assigning causal explanations for problems to individual differences or to the culture, however, it turns out not to be simple. Each individual belongs simultaneously to concentric and intersecting subcultures, defined by the nation, the ethnic group, the era, the neighbourhood, the peer group, the work group, and the family. Each subculture may have its own rules with respect to substance use. Since these rules can conflict, following the rules of one subculture may lead to problems defined by another without any individual contribution at all, as when the unlucky 17–year-old is arrested for drinking, although 90 per cent of his peers also do so.

Since rule violation alone is not evidence for individual causal factors, we must look for other criteria. One possibility would be to divide the correlates of substance abuse into those that are cultural and those that are individual. Unfortunately, most of the variables known to be correlated with substance abuse problems can be either. Age, for example, is both an indicator of the individual's developmental status and an indicator of the likely values of his peer group. Similarly, with gender; if women have fewer substance use problems than men, it is not obvious whether female hormones protect them from adverse reactions to drugs, or whether cultural patterns that introduce women to substances later than men and more severely limit the quantities they ingest are responsible. Thus, we cannot sort the correlates of substance use problems into cultural and individual sets.

There are certain strategies, however, that can be helpful. Correlates that can predict which of a pair of siblings reared together will develop substance abuse are likely to be individual variables, because siblings share so many of their cultural spheres, although even they do not grow up in identical eras unless they are twins and even then may not share peer groups. Geneticists have devised a variety of designs to tease apart genetic from environmental determinants, using special samples of twins and cross-fostered children. While they thus identify genetic endowment, *one* individual factor, their designs cannot separate non-genetic individual variation from extra-familial cultural effects.

We suggest here a strategy that is also imperfect, but which goes some way toward detecting individual differences. It also has the advantage of being usable in general population samples, not solely in samples known to share genes. We focus on predictors that those with substantial use of substances will develop problems, rather than looking at predictors of abuse in the population as a whole. This strategy grows out of thinking of the development of substance abuse problems as a passage through three gates: first use, then use at a rate high enough to create a reasonable risk of problems, then the development of a problem. There is also a fourth gate, which is persistence in use once a problem is recognized. When use is quickly dropped or severely reduced once a problem occurs, the problem is almost never brought to public attention, and may not even be thought worth reporting by the person briefly experiencing it. Thus we are, in fact, only able to predict which substantial users will develop *persistent* problems.

Because culture regulates what substances to use, when to use them, and how much to use, it plays a major role, along with individual factors, in the passage through the first two gates: deciding whether to use and whether to use heavily enough to create the potential for problems. A substance use problem (or substance abuse), however, can be defined as substance use at a level or in a way that 'produces behaviour changes (that) would be viewed as extremely undesirable in almost all cultures' (American Psychiatric Association 1987). Because passing through the fourth gate (the transformation of heavy use into recognized problem use) is generally not culturally sanctioned, it must usually be explained by individual variation. Of course, the individual variations may themselves by created by the culture (e.g. high levels of anxiety may be caused by attending a highly competitive school), but we count as cultural determinants only cultural norms specific to substance use. The one case where culture appears to be a proximal cause of problems is when individuals belong simultaneously to cultures with conflicting norms concerning substance abuse. Thus, social problems occur when teetotaling parents complain about children's levels of drinking that are acceptable in the wider culture. Granting this and other possible exceptions, the transition from heavy drinking to problems is *more* likely to be explained by individual variation than are the other transitions along the path to problems, from non-use to use or from very occasional to regular use.

Unfortunately, the literature available for pursuing this strategy is limited. Most studies provide correlates only of quantity and frequency of use or only of problems. Results from the few studies that have collected information on both quantity/frequency and problems are not always published in a form in which problem rates can be calculated for the subsample of users as well as for the total population.

Because heavy users are a relatively small proportion of the population, unless the study is done in a high risk population, samples must be large to provide the necessary data. A study which provides information about both heavy use of alcohol and drugs and problems associated with them, is the Epidemiologic Catchment Area project (ECA), a survey carried out between 1980 and 1983 with some 20 000 American adults of all ages in five geographic areas. It can tell us what proportion of a general population passes through our gates of use, heavy use, and problem use, and their probabilities of transition to problems at each point. Thirty per cent had used some illicit drug, passing the first gate. Heavy drug use, defined as daily use for at least two weeks, occurred in 8 per cent, and 6 per cent had sufficient problems to qualify for a DSM-III diagnosis of drug abuse or dependence (Anthony et al. 1991). The likelihood of transition from use to problems was 31 per cent; from daily use to problems, 54 per cent.

For alcohol, use was defined as ever taking a drink on one's own, and two levels of heavy drinking were defined: seven or more drinks per occasion at least once a week for several months, and seven or more drinks daily for at least two weeks. Alcohol problems, like drug problems, were defined as meeting DSM-III criteria for abuse or dependence. Almost the whole population (89 per cent) had used alcohol, about one-quarter (23 per cent) had drunk heavily weekly, 7 per cent had been daily heavy drinkers, and 14 per cent met criteria for abuse or dependence (Helzer et al. 1991). Weekly heavy drinking was a nearly necessary condition to the development of problems, and heavy daily drinking was a nearly sufficient condition. Among those who drank but never heavily, only 5 per cent qualified as having problems, among those who drank heavily weekly but never daily, 43 per cent had problems, and among those who were daily heavy drinkers, 91 per cent had problems.

AVAILABLE VARIABLES

Within appropriate studies we have found the following correlates that can be examined with regard to the point in the transition to problems at which they have an impact: (1) familial substance abuse, (2) gender, (3) age, (4) ethnicity, (5) childhood behaviour, (6) adult psychiatric disorder, and (7) life events. We will review available studies with respect to these variables, and add newly analysed data from the ECA to amplify the existing data sets.

Biological correlates have also been studied. However, to distinguish biological predispositions in which we are interested from biological phenomena which are the *effects* of substances on the system, biological characteristics must be evaluated prior to beginning substance use, and subjects followed to see which pre-existing biological characteristics predict substance use problems. But what should be measured? A necessary first step to allow choosing relevant variables is to look for biological abnormalities in offspring of abusers still too young to have begun use as, for example, Begleiter *et al.* (1984) have done. The follow-ups to see whether these differences in fact predict vulnerability have yet to be completed.

FINDINGS

1. Familial substance abuse

Parental alcohol problems meet our criteria as indicators of individual liability. Not only do children of inadequate and alcoholic parents have more alcohol problems than others, but *among heavy drinkers* they more often develop problems (Robins *et al.* 1991; Reich *et al.* 1975; Vaillant 1983; McCord 1990). We cannot say as much about the role of drug use and abuse in the parental generation because few older people have used illicit drugs, not having been personally affected by the drug epidemic that began in the 1960s and affected mainly young adults. None the less, several studies have shown that the presence of drug abuse as well as alcoholism in first degree relatives increases the chance that drug use will progress to problem use (Stiffman *et al.* 1987; Cadoret *et al.* 1980).

In the ECA, family psychiatric history was not routinely obtained, but the St Louis site investigated it in the second wave. This much smaller sample included few reports of drug abusing parents. We therefore combined those abusing alcohol or drugs. Effects of parental abuse were greater on heavy *use* than on the transition from heavy use to problems (see Table 8.1, bottom panel), although there is a trend toward more problems among heavy users when parents were abusers.

The propensity for those who use substances heavily to develop problems when their parents have problems suggests that there may be a genetic liability. Another possibility is an effect of living in a family where drinking is part of the culture. For example, when parents are substance abusers,

TABLE 8.1 Correlates of heavy use and correlates of problems among heavy users (in per cent in 4 ECA sites — St Louis, Baltimore, Los Angeles, Durham, both interviews)

		Alcohol		Drugs	
		Heavy use	Problems among heavy users	Heavy use	Problems among heavy users
Demographics					
Sex	Male	28	76	13	50
	Female	6***	57***	6***	51
Age	18–29	17	70	20	51
	30–44	18	72	12***	49
	45–64	13**	73	1***	55
	65+	9***	70	0	-
Ethnic	White	16	70	10	52
group	Black	11**	82	8	42
	Hispanic	13	81	6	50
High risk group for heavy use:					
Whites below age 45					
	Male	32	76	23	52
	Female	9	51	12	51
Residence in 'dry' area					
	Durham, NC	9	73	5	48
	Elsewhere	16***	74	10***	49

Childhood history				
Age of first use				
Below 15	45	78	68	64
Later	12***	69*	8***	48**
Behaviour problems before 15				
<2	10	65	6	42
2	30**	70	19***	52
3–4	42***	81†††	30***	64†††
5+	65***	94**	50**	63‡‡
Preceding psychiatric symptoms				
Manic or psychotic before first problem				
No	15	71	9	49
Yes	41***	88*	39***	80***
Depression before first problem				
No	15	72	9	49
Yes	15	62	13*	63*
'Nervous' before first problem				
No	15	70	9	46
Yes	16	74	11	66***
Family history (St Louis second wave only)				
Parental substance abuse				
No	15	68	7	51
Yes	32***	81	18***	59

* = Significant difference from next level up; † = significant difference from 2 levels up; ‡ = significant difference from 3 levels up; 1 symbols = $p < .05$; 2 symbols = $p < .01$; 3 symbols = $p < .001$.

their children are likely to be exposed to alcohol very early, as compared to children in other families, who generally wait until their peers begin to drink. As we shall see below, early use may create individual propensities to problem use.

A definitive separation of genetic from environmental effects of family substance abuse requires studies of cross-fostering or of identical vs fraternal twins. These studies have indicated some genetic contribution to at least some types of substance abuse (Cloninger *et al.* 1981; Goodwin *et al.* 1973; Schuckit *et al.* 1972; Cadoret *et al.* 1986). Unfortunately these studies rarely report on both heavy drinking and problem drinking. However, Goodwin *et al.* (1973) did find that male adoptees who were heavy drinkers were more likely to develop problems if they had an alcoholic biological parent (55 per cent vs 35 per cent).

Major efforts funded by NIAAA are underway to try to identify the gene or genes responsible for familial transmission of alcohol dependence.

2. Gender

The ECA results show that male alcoholics outnumber females by about 5 to 1, and that drug abuse is almost twice as common in men as women. But a large part of this difference is explained by the fact that fewer men than women abstain entirely, and that men who drink begin use younger and use alcohol and drugs more heavily than do female drinkers. As Table 8.1 shows, 28 per cent of men vs 6 per cent of women were heavy drinkers, 13 per cent of men and 6 per cent of women were substantial drug users. Among heavy drinkers in the ECA, more men than women met criteria for an alcohol disorder: 76 per cent vs 57 per cent of women. While according to our strategy this would suggest that gender itself is an individual factor in alcohol problems, it may only be cultural — reflecting the fact that men begin drinking heavily earlier than women. Men who ever drank enough to get drunk did so first at an average age of 15.1 years. For women ever drunk, the first time was about a year and a half later (16.6 years of age). For drugs, the gender difference is entirely explained by more males using heavily (13 per cent vs 6 per cent); among heavy drug users, there was no sex difference in rate of problems (50 per cent of males, 51 per cent of females). This similarity is consistent with finding minimal differences in the ages at which men and women began illicit drug use — they differed by only 3 months. However, later first use of drugs by young women was reported in New York blacks (Brunswick 1978).

The finding that gender differences were more probably cultural than biological was first noted in our follow up of child guidance clinic patients (Robins *et al.* 1991). The three-fold difference in alcoholism between male and female ex-patients (21 per cent vs 8 per cent) dropped to insignificance

Detecting individual factors in substance abuse problems 141

(57 per cent vs 44 per cent) among those who drank heavily. Similar results were found among New York youngsters (Brunswick 1978).

3. Age

The prevalence of substance abuse has risen enormously over the last 50 years, with the end of Prohibition and the beginning of a drug epidemic. These historic changes have primarily affected younger cohorts. It appears that the maximum intake of substances is typically in early adulthood, and that changes in availability thereafter have little effect.

That the inverse correlation of substance abuse with age is cultural rather than individual is shown in a study by Cahalan and Room (1972), of a national sample of men. While young men (under 30) were twice as likely to have drinking problems as men aged 50–59 (21 per cent vs 11 per cent), this was explained by there being fewer abstainers and more heavy drinkers among the young. Among heavy drinkers, rates of problems were comparable across all age groups.

In the ECA (Table 8.1), the proportion of ever heavy drinkers was higher in those under 45 (18 per cent), than in those 45–64 (13 per cent) or over 65 (9 per cent). But there was *no* age effect in proportion with problems among heavy drinkers. Similarly, there was a striking effect of age on heavy drug use, with almost no heavy users above age 45, but no effects of age on problems among users.

The lack of individual effects of age may be surprising, since biological effects of age seem paramount in explaining why older alcoholics have often terminated their heavy drinking and drug use. Old people may develop illnesses for which drinking is contra-indicated, or require medications with which alcohol and drugs should not be combined, or experience adverse effects as the rapidity with which the body can metabolize alcohol and drugs declines. But the contributions of the biological effects of age to *terminating* problems obviously would not influence whether problems will have occurred when the person was younger. Age as related to *lifetime* substance use problems reflects the historic period in which one grew up, not the developmental stage at interview.

One of the most striking and well-replicated effects of age is that early introduction to drinking and drugs predicts that problems will develop. Earlier alcohol or drug use was associated with more problems for both male and female New York youth (Brunswick 1978), for Swedish men born in a single year (Andersson and Magnusson 1988), for black men born between 1931 and 1935 and growing up in St Louis (Robins and Murphy 1967), for Vietnam veterans returning in 1971 (Robins *et al.* 1980), for St Louis ECA drug users under age 35 (Robins and Przybeck 1985), and for the total ECA sample of drug users.

Among ECA drug users, men who first used drugs before age 15 developed problems in 51 per cent of cases, compared with 16 per cent who began at 18 or later. Comparable figures for women are 39 per cent developing problems if they began drug use before 15, and 12 per cent if they were over 18. We considered the possibility that this effect of age merely resulted from earlier use when children had more predictors of drug problems. Deviant childhood behaviour (see below) did predict early use as well as problems with substances. However, holding level of behaviour problems constant, age of first use still had an independent effect (Robins and McEvoy 1990).

These published results showed that age of onset affected rate of problems among users, but this effect might have been only through increasing the number who use *heavily*. However, among *heavy* users, those beginning use before 15 were significantly more likely to develop problems with both alcohol and drugs than those beginning later (Table 8.1). Thus early use is likely to be either an *indicator* of individual differences associated with later problems *or* to be the cause of an increase in the individual's problem-proneness.

4. Ethnicity

Like age and sex, ethnicity has both cultural and biological aspects. Culturally, it is strongly linked to membership in particular religions, which may forbid use of psychoactive substances or may require it as part of their rites. Because of endogamy over many generations, ethnic groups also have some degree of biological homogeneity; they also share eating patterns and often place of residence and work place, and so share culturally determined similarities in their biology that may affect their reactions to psychoactive drugs.

Sociologists in the 1940s paid considerable attention to cultural aspects of ethnic differences in drinking problems. Americans of Irish background were found to have particularly high rates of alcohol problems, and Jews to have particularly low rates. Explanations were sought in the different meanings attached to drinking in these cultures. In a follow-up of child guidance clinic patients (Robins *et al.* 1991), the expected high rates of alcohol problems in those of Irish extraction and low rates in Jews were found. This study substantiated the interpretation that this was more likely a cultural than a biological phenomenon because among *heavy drinkers*, there was no difference between Irish and Jews in proportions developing problems. The difference in their rates of drinking problems was entirely explained by the larger proportion of heavy drinkers among Irish men.

The drinking minority in 'dry' areas of the US, where fundamentalist religions are common, were reported to have a particular liability to develop problems (Cahalan and Room 1972). This could have had either cultural or individual explanations: abstinent cultures do not provide norms for how much and how rapidly to drink, and so do not teach moderate drinking — a cultural explanation. On the other hand, persons with psychological needs for alcohol that predict problem drinking, might constitute the majority of the drinkers in an abstinent culture, because those who would elsewhere drink for sociability or celebration would abstain, having no drinking peers with whom to socialize or celebrate — an individual liability explanation.

More recent studies do not confirm the earlier results; while the proportion of heavy drinkers is much lower in the 'Bible belt' than elsewhere in the US, among heavy drinkers, location does not predict the proportion who will develop problems (Helzer *et al.* 1991, and Table 8.1). This is likely a historic change; with increased geographic mobility, the traditionally 'dry' areas have been infiltrated by drinkers. These newcomers, plus the waning power of fundamentalist religions, result in a majority of the population being drinkers even in the 'driest' areas.

The ECA found drinking problems to be more common among Mexican-American than white men but less common among Mexican-American than white women (Helzer *et al.* 1991). As a consequence, the ratio of male to female problem drinkers is especially large for Mexican-Americans. As compared with whites, black male to female ratios of alcohol abuse were small (Robins *et al.* 1980) and overall, blacks were the group with the smallest proportion of heavy drinkers. Among heavy drinkers, there were no statistically significant ethnic differences in rate of problems (Table 8.1). For drug use, no significant ethnic differences were found either in rates of heavy use *or* in rates of problem use among heavy users. For alcohol problems (but not drugs), however, blacks' cohort patterns differed from whites': for whites, lifetime problem rates were inversely related to age, while for blacks, age and problems were unrelated. Thus *older* blacks include more substance abusers than same-aged whites, while *younger* blacks include fewer.

The smaller contrast by age groups in blacks than whites with respect to problem drinking in the US is most likely an effect of historic events. Sixty years ago, most blacks in the US lived in the rural South and were adherents of the abstinent religions of those areas. Around the Second World War, great numbers left the South for the northern and midwestern cities where defence jobs offered improved living standards. With the strict controls of rural Baptist cultures loosened, the immigrants began not only to drink and use drugs, but displayed in the high rate of pathological use described by Cahalan and Room among drinkers from abstinent cultures. Those immigrants are now the grandparents and ageing parents of young adult urban blacks. In the young adult generation, the earlier pattern seems to be re-emerging, resulting in lower rates than for young whites. National surveys of levels of use also find black rates of heavy use higher than whites' in the older population, and lower than whites' among the young. Because this ethnic pattern is found at the level of heavy use as well as problems, it is more likely to be a cultural than an individual variable.

In a study of Vietnam veterans who had been addicted while in Vietnam (Robins *et al.* 1980), blacks who used narcotics after return in 1971 to 1973 were less likely than whites to become re-addicted. This seems likely a mix of cultural and individual phenomena, explainable by the greater use of heroin in the inner city than in the suburbs. Presumably white users, who were using narcotic drugs in a setting of relative scarcity, like drinkers in abstinent cultures of the 1960s, were driven to use by individual needs, while a proportion of blacks were motivated by simple sociability. This interpretation is supported by the finding in a study of adolescents attending inner city clinics, that both use of alcohol and drugs and problems with them were more common in whites than blacks (Stiffman *et al.* 1987). White adolescents attending the free inner city clinics that cater primarily to black adolescents were largely youngsters who had broken off relationships with their parents; they had a high rate of a variety of social and psychiatric problems, that probably predisposed them to use of drugs and to the development of problems if they used. In cultures in which use is rare and disapproved, only the more deviant become users, resulting in a high proportion of problems among users.

5. Childhood behaviour and emotional problems

While most substance abusers do not have a history of conduct disorder in childhood, the risk for abuse among children with behaviour problems is extraordinarily high. In the ECA, the impact of childhood behaviour problems was found at multiple points in the transition to problem use: conduct problems were associated with more use of illicit substances, with a lower age at which substance use would be initiated, with increased likelihood that use would be heavy, and with a greater risk that heavy users would become problem users (Table 8.1). The impact of conduct problems on substance use problems was experienced by both early and late initiators of substance use (Robins and McEvoy 1990). Other studies substantiate these findings. In our study of young black men (Robins *et al.* 1968), behaviour problems measured by failure and absence in elementary schools, failure to complete high school, and delinquency, not only predicted heavy drinking, but that heavy drinkers would develop alcohol problems. Indeed, less than half the heavy drinkers who finished high school after an uneventful elementary school career developed any problems, while almost all (94 per cent) heavy drinkers who had become delinquent at age 15 or 16 and failed to graduate developed problems with alcohol. Similarly, among those who ever used heroin, 94 per cent of the delinquents became addicted, compared with 54 per cent of the non-delinquents (Robins and Murphy 1967).

In addition to prior delinquent behaviour, low self esteem and anti-establishment attitudes have been found to be related to substance abuse. In an analysis of a Los Angeles follow-up study of school children, drug and alcohol problems in young adulthood were predicted by adolescent delinquent behaviour, left-wing politics, and self-derogation, even after controlling for frequency of use (Newcomb and Bentler 1990).

In the study of adolescents attending inner-city clinics (Stiffman *et al.* 1987), those abusing drugs exceeded those who used without problems in symptoms of anxiety, depression, suicidal ideation, and conduct disorder.

6. Adult personality and psychiatric disorder

The link between substance abuse problems and adult behaviours such as fighting, crime, and marital conflicts are so well known that there is no need to reiterate them here. There are two plausible alternatives to the belief that these behaviours indicate a predisposition to substance abuse: (1) the adult antisocial behaviour and the drug problems may have common roots in childhood behaviour problems without being causally connected to each other, or (2) the substance abuse may cause adult antisocial behaviour. Because adult antisocial behaviour and substance abuse occur in the same time period, it is difficult to separate cause from effect. In principle, onsets of both the adult behaviours and the transition from heavy substance use to problems could be dated to help determine which is cart and which horse, but we found no study that had actually dated both.

We know a little more about the contribution of the abuse of one type of substance to the abuse of another. From the ECA data, we were able to construct a scale of the types of substances with which problems were experienced. This scale replicated a scale of substance *use* constructed for New York high school students (Yamaguchi and Kandel 1985). Further, it met criteria for a Guttman Scale in every one of the 5 ECA settings (Robins and McEvoy 1990). A Guttman scale implies that the items occurred in temporal sequence. Thus, our scale implies that alcohol problems precede problems with marijuana, which in turn precede problems with stimulants, tranquillizers, and sedatives, and these in turn precede problems with opiates and cocaine. While temporal precedence does not prove that problems with one drug increases the predisposition to problems with another, it is consistent with this hypothesis. We know that there are important cultural factors in the progression from *use* of one drug to *use* of another.

Users tend to find friends among other users and to turn their drug-naïve friends into users. This circle of friends then provides access to, and companions-in-use of, drugs not yet tried. The mechanisms for progression from *problems* with one drug to *problems* with another have not been established. Further studies are needed to learn whether earlier problems with one drug create a vulnerability to problems with a drug of a different type.

There is a striking relationship between substance abuse and certain psychiatric disorders. In the ECA, the odds ratios for the association between drug or alcohol abuse and other disorders are highest with antisocial personality, and next highest with mania and schizophrenia (Helzer and Przybeck 1988; Anthony *et al.* 1991). Table 8.1 shows that mania and psychotic symptoms were both followed by an increase both in using heavily and in heavy users developing problems with alcohol and other drugs. In contrast, prior depression and nervousness did not increase the risk of either heavy drinking or the development of alcohol problems among heavy drinkers. Depression, however, was associated with heavy drug use, and both depression and nervousness were frequently followed by drug problems among heavy users.

7. Life events

Although both cultural membership and individual predispositions affect the chances of experiencing particular life events, it is widely believed that life events can create changes in individual predispositions. The Vietnam study provided an opportunity to see how experiencing one major life event — going to war in a strange country where heroin and morphine were at least as available as alcohol — affected alcohol (Wish *et al.* 1979) and drug problems (Robins *et al.* 1980). As compared with civilians identified in Selective Service records and matched to the veterans for age, education, and eligibility for service, the veterans showed much the greater changes in their drug and alcohol use and in substance-related problems during the year in which they were in Vietnam. Indeed, their level of heroin addiction in Vietnam was more than 20 times that of the civilian comparison group during the equivalent year. But the effects of drug use in the military were transitory, while the effects of their pre-service behaviour problems and substance use were not. After the first year back from Vietnam, pre-military behaviour, including arrests, school dropout, fighting, and heavy alcohol and drug use, was as strongly associated with current use and abuse of substances in veterans as in non-veterans, and absolute levels of use and problems among veterans were the same as among civilians once differences in pre-service behaviours were taken into account.

CONCLUSIONS

We noted that correlates of substance abuse are not easily distinguished as being individual or cultural factors, or a mixture of the two. None the less, there are both theoretical and practical reasons for wanting to identify factors that have at least some individual component. Theoretically, the existence of individual variables is consistent with the medical model, i.e. that substance abuse disorders are real, although it does not prove it. Practically, individual variables suggest target populations for intervention and may suggest interventions to be offered, while cultural variables would seem to require more society-wide plans.

We have argued that factors that are correlated with problems only because they predict who will use substances at a frequency and quantity high enough to make problems a possibility, and do not predict who among those substantially exposed will develop problems, may well be cultural rather than individual variables. Variables that predict movement from heavy to problem use appear more likely to be individual than cultural variables, because cultures do not support such transitions. We have reviewed the somewhat sparse literature that allows this discrimination, and have supplemented it with analyses from the Epidemiologic Catchment Area project.

Among the variables we have considered, birth cohort (age), gender, residence in dry areas, and ethnicity appear to be primarily cultural factors. Childhood behaviour problems, early exposure to substances, and parental substance abuse appear to be indicators of individual vulnerability, because they predict transition from heavy to problem use. However, they may be indicators of cultural factors as well, because they also predict who will become a heavy user. Prior psychiatric disorders are probably exclusively individual variables, because there is no subculture of schizophrenics, manics, depressives, or 'nervous' people. A major life event, service in the Vietnam war, was shown to have remarkably little ability to permanently deflect individual and cultural differences established in adolescence once men returned to the US.

If our conclusions are correct, we need to consider through what mechanisms parental substance abuse, early exposure to substances, childhood behaviour problems, and psychiatric symptoms create such individual predispositions to substance abuse problems. Psychiatric disorders may have various effects: first, their symptoms, including anxiety, restlessness, and intrusive thoughts, may inspire self-medication with drugs and alcohol. Second, they may impair the user's 'reality testing', i.e. his ability to perceive his increasing dependence or the social disapproval of his excessive use, and so prevent his stopping in time to prevent problems.

Third, they may impair his ability to modify his behaviour when he does recognize that he is in difficulty. Fourth, he may fail to stop use when problems arise because he misattributes his difficulties to the psychiatric disorder rather than to his substance use. Finally, his illness may have isolated him from his peers, so that they are not available to apply the social controls that more normal substance users experience.

Unlike those with adult psychiatric disorders, children with conduct problems do tend to develop delinquent subcultures that can encourage early use of drugs and heavy use. Much has been written about the pro-drug and -alcohol norms of delinquent peers, and the opportunities they provide for participating in substance use. However, the fact that those with a history of conduct problems progress easily from heavy to problem use, may reflect their own personalities rather than the impact of their peer group. Recklessness, boredom, and a tendency to value present gratification over future goals may explain why they do not restrict their use at the first sign of difficulties, as their temperamentally more cautious and less impulsive age peers do.

Early exposure to substances is much influenced by family and peer cultures. None the less, from the fact that heavy users exposed early more frequently develop problems, we argue that whatever the reason it happens, early exposure appears to increase the individual's susceptibility to develop problems. One mechanism might be that immature nervous systems may be permanently affected by psychoactive substances. Such vulnerabilities have been reported in animals. Animal models would appear to be the logical starting point for searching for critical developmental periods, during which there is a risk of long-lasting damage from drugs and alcohol.

Our argument that variables that influence the transition from heavy use to problem use are likely to be individual variables has not yet been proved correct. Proof requires experiments in modifying these variables or their consequences at the individual level, to see whether the burden of substance abuse problems is thus reduced. But the segregation of predictors according to *which* transitions on the path to problems they affect, may be useful even before we have such proof. Variables that have their chief impact in predicting heavy use are candidates for early interventions with non-users and casual users, perhaps through community-wide programmes; interventions involving variables that affect transition from heavy use to problems are appropriate for implementation through outreach programmes designed to identify heavy users before they develop problems.

REFERENCES

American Psychiatric Association (1987). *Diagnostic and statistical manual* (3rd ed., revised). American Psychiatric Association Press, Washington, DC.

Andersson, T. and Magnusson, D. (1988). Drinking habits and alcohol abuse among young men: a prospective longitudinal study. *Journal of Studies on Alcohol*, **49**, 245–52.

Anthony, J. A., Helzer J. E., and McEvoy, L. T. (1991). Syndromes of drug use and dependence. In Robins, L. N. and Regier, D. A. (eds), *Psychiatric disorders in America* pp. 116–54. The Free Press, New York.

Begleiter, H., Porjesz, B., Bihari, B., and Kissin, B. (1984). Event regulated brain potentials in boys at risk for alcoholism. *Science*, **225**, 1493–6.

Brunswick, A. (1978). *Black youth and drug use behavior*. Mimeograph, (unpublished).

Cadoret, R. J., Can, C. A., and Grove, W. M. (1980). Development of alcoholism in adoptees raised apart from alcoholic biologic relatives. *Archives of General Psychiatry*, **37**, 561–3.

Cadoret, R. J., O'Gorman, T. W., Heywood, E., and Troughton, E. (1986). An adoption study of genetic and environmental factors in drug abuse. *Archives of General Psychiatry*, **43**, 1131–6.

Cahalan, D. and Room, R. (1972). Problem drinking among American men aged 21–59. *American Journal of Public Health*, **62**, 1473–82.

Cloninger, C. R., Bohman, M., and Sigvardsson, S. (1981). Inheritance of alcohol abuse: cross-fostering analysis of adopted men. *Archives of General Psychiatry*, **38**, 861–8.

Fillmore, K. M. (1987). Prevalence, incidence and chronicity of drinking patterns and problems among men as a function of age: a longitudinal and cohort analysis. *British Journal of Addiction*, **82**, 77–83.

Goodwin, D. W., Schulsinger, F., Moller N, Hermansen, L., Winokur, G., and Guze, S. B. (1973). Alcohol problems in adoptees raised apart from biological parents. *Archives of General Psychiatry*, **28**, 238–43.

Helzer, J. E. and Przybeck, T. R. (1988). The co-occurrence of alcoholism and other psychiatric disorder in the general population and its impact on treatment. *Journal of Studies on Alcohol*, **49**, 219–24.

Helzer, J. E. and Robins, L. N. (1985). Specification of predictors of narcotic use versus addiction. In Robins, L. N. (ed.), *Studying drug use and abuse*. Series in Psychosocial Epidemiology, No. 6 (ed. A. E. Slaby), pp. 173–97. Rutgers University Press, New Brunswick.

Helzer, J. E., Burnam, A., and McEvoy, L. T. (1991). Alcohol abuse and dependence. In Robins, L. N., and Regier, D. A. (eds), *Psychiatric disorders in America*, pp. 81–115. The Free Press, New York.

King, L. J., Murphy, G. E., Robins, L. N., and Darvish, H. (1969). Alcohol abuse: a crucial factor in the social problems of Negro men. *American Journal of Psychiatry*, **125**, 1682–90.

McCord, J. (1990). Long-term perspectives on parental absence. In Robins, L. N. and Rutter, M. (eds), *Straight and devious pathways from childhood to adulthood* pp. 116–34. Cambridge University Press, Cambridge.

Newcomb, M. D., and Bentler, P. M. (1990). Antecedents and consequences of cocaine use: an eight-year study from early adolescence to young adulthood. In *Straight and devious pathways from childhood to adulthood* Robins, L., and Rutter, M. (eds), pp. 158–81. Cambridge University Press, Cambridge.

Reich, R., Winokur, G., and Mullaney, J. (1975). The transmission of alcoholism. In Fieve, R. F., Rosenthal, D., and Brill H. (eds), *Genetic research in psychiatry*, Proceedings of the 63rd Meeting of the American Psychopathological Association, 1973, pp. 259–71. Johns Hopkins Press, Baltimore.

Robins, L. N. (1989). Alcohol abuse in blacks and whites as indicated in the Epidemiological Catchment Area Program. In Spiegler, D., Tate, D. A., Aitken, S. S., and Christian, C. M. (eds). *Alcohol use among us ethnic minorities*, NIAAA Research Monograph No. 18, DHHS Pub. No. (ADM 88–1435), Washington, DC.

Robins, L. N., Bates, W. M., and O'Neal, P. (1991). Adult drinking patterns of former problem children. In Pittman, D. J., and White, H. (eds), *Society, culture, and drinking patterns, re-examined*, pp. 460–79, Rutger Center of Alcohol Studies, New Burnswick, New Jersey.

Robins, L. N. and McEvoy, L. T. (1990). Conduct problems as predictors of substance abuse. In Robins, L. N., and Rutter, M. (eds), *Straight and devious pathways from childhood to adulthood*, pp. 182–204. Cambridge University Press, Cambridge.

Robins, L. N. and Murphy, G. E. (1967). Drug use in a normal population of young Negro men. *American Journal of Public Health*, **57**, 1580–96.

Robins, L. N. and Przybeck, T. R. (1985). Age of onset of drug use as a factor in drug and other disorders. In Jones, C. L. and Battjes, R. J. (eds), *Etiology of drug abuse: implications for prevention*, NIDA Research Monograph 56, DHHS Publication No. (ADM 85–1335), pp. 178–92. Washington, DC.

Robins, L. N., Murphy, G. E., and Breckenridge, M. B. (1968). Drinking behavior of young urban Negro men. *Quarterly Journal of Studies on Alcohol*, **29**, 657–84.

Robins, L. N., Helzer, J. E., Hesselbrock, M., and Wish, E. (1980). Vietnam veterans three years after Vietnam. In Brill, L. and Winick, C. (eds), *Yearbook of substance use and abuse*, pp. 213–30. Human Sciences Press, New York.

Schuckit, M. A., Goodwin, D. W., and Winokur, G. (1972). A study of alcoholism in half-siblings. *American Journal of Psychiatry*, **128**, 1132–5.

Stiffman, A. R., Earls F., Powell, J., and Robins, L. N. (1987). Correlates of alcohol and illicit drug use in adolescent medical patients. *Contemporary Drug Problems*, Summer, 295–314.

Vaillant, G. E. (1983). *The natural history of alcoholism*. Harvard University Press, Cambridge, Massachusetts.

Wish, E., Robins, L., Hesselbrock, M., and Helzer, J. (1979). The course of alcohol problems in Vietnam veterans. In Galanter, M. (ed), *Currents in alcoholism*, pp. 239–56. Grune and Stratton, New York.

Yamaguchi, K. and Kandel, D. B. (1984). Patterns of drug use from adolescence to young adulthood. II. Sequences of progression. *American Journal of Public Health*, **74**, 668–71.

9

Individual susceptibility to alcohol abuse and to ethanol toxicity

TIMOTHY J. PETERS

One of the most interesting challenges concerning alcohol abuse and toxicity is the basis for the individual susceptibility to abuse, dependency, and selective organ toxicity. Thus, only 5 per cent of alcohol consumers become alcohol abusers and of these only 20 per cent develop cirrhosis. Although amount of alcohol consumption and the pattern of drinking are important determinants of alcohol dependency and tissue damage, these cannot alone explain either the clinical or pathological consequences in individual subjects. Another related area of interest is the question of the differential gender and racial susceptibility to toxicity. These vary markedly between different racial groups and between men and women and, again, are not closely related to overall consumption.

This review attempts to address some of these questions using selected examples to illustrate the underlying principles. A brief account of the key pathways of alcohol metabolism is provided. Ethanol is principally metabolized in the liver by alcohol dehydrogenase (ADH) to yield the potentially toxic intermediate acetaldehyde (Fig. 9.1). This is further metabolized by acetaldehyde dehydrogenases (ALDH) to the metabolic fuel acetate. ADH is present solely in the soluble fraction of the cell and ALDH is found in both the soluble fraction and the mitochondria (the principle energy supplier). As side reactions of this pathway, various complex metabolic reactions in the cell are interfered with and, in addition, free radicals and reactive oxygen species are formed. These potentially highly-toxic, short-lived molecules can damage most biological molecules, including DNA, lipids, proteins, carbohydrates, and low molecular weight compounds (Halliwell and Gutteridge 1985).

They are normally produced by several biological reactions, but formation is markedly increased in a variety of disorders, including alcohol abuse. Cells and most body fluids contain a variety of free radical scavengers, e.g. glutathione, α-tocopherol (vitamin E), and superoxide dismutase, which limit the toxic effects of these reactive oxygen species.

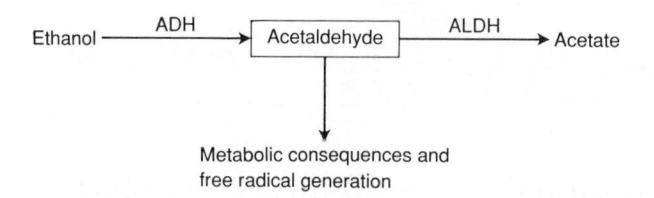

152 *The Nature of Alcohol and Drug Related Problems*

```
Ethanol ──ADH──▶ [Acetaldehyde] ──ALDH──▶ Acetate
                      │
                      ▼
              Metabolic consequences and
              free radical generation
```

FIG. 9.1 Principal pathway of ethanol metabolism.

ETHNIC VARIATIONS

Much of the evidence is anecdotal or has not been subjected to critical and case-controlled analysis. However, certain information is consistent and for some ethnic groups resistance (aversion) to alcohol is well-documented (Wolff 1972; Ewing *et al.* 1974; Wilson *et al.* 1978). It is well known that certain Oriental subjects show a reduced susceptibility to developing alcohol abuse (Table 9.1), and this has been closely correlated with a response to alcohol of an intense unpleasant facial flushing associated with autonomic effects (Goedde and Agarwal 1987). Recently, the basis for this reaction has been defined in molecular terms. A single nucleotide-base change in the subjects' DNA sequence coding for acetaldehyde dehydrogenase leads to a glutamate to lysine substitution in the mitochondrial enzyme (Yoshida *et al.* 1984). Although the enzyme protein is present in these subjects, often in increased amounts, the protein exhibits no enzymatic activity so that, after a modest dose of ethanol, markedly (10-fold) increased blood levels of acetaldehyde are found causing the intensely aversive effects in these subjects (Mizoi *et al.* 1979) (Table 9.2). The abnormality is inherited as a dominant trait (Goedde and Agarwal 1987). Recent studies of genotyping, i.e. studying the structure of their relevant genes, control subjects and patients with alcoholic liver disease, have confirmed the protective effect of this genetic defect against the development of alcoholism, and alcoholic liver disease in particular. There was no association of alcoholic liver disease with the genotype of alcohol dehydrogenases (Shibuya and Yoshida 1988).

Recently, we have investigated some Caucasian subjects who exhibit a flush reaction after consuming small amounts of alcohol (Yoshida *et al.* 1989). This phenomenon is anecdotally well-recognized, but has been little studied. Our studies indicate a prevalence of flushing in Caucasians, particularly female subjects, of approximately 20 per cent (Ward and Peters, unpublished results). Three such subjects have been identified with reduced red blood cell acetaldehyde dehydrogenase activity. In one family studied in detail, inheritance appears to be as a dominant trait with variable expression (Peters *et al.* 1990). Interestingly, the grandfathers of the subject were

TABLE 9.1 *Distribution of mitochondrial acetaldehyde dehydrogenase variants in Japanese subjects*

Patient group	Variant (%)	
	Normal	Inactive
Normal subjects (105)	59	41
Alcoholics (175)	98	2
Drug addicts (47)	51	49
Schizophrenics (86)	58	42

Number of subjects shown between parentheses. Data from Goedde and Agarwal (1987).

TABLE 9.2 *Peak blood ethanol and aetaldehyde levels in normal and acetaldehyde dehydrogenase variant Japanese after an ethanol test dose*

ALDH	Ethanol (mmol l^{-1})	Acetaldehyde (μmol l^{-1})
Normal	10.3 ± 1.9	2.1 ± 1.7
Variant	10.9 ± 2.3	35.4 ± 12.8

Mean ± SD peak blood levels after 0.4 g kg^{-1} body weight of ethanol. Results reproduced from Goedde and Agarwal (1987).

alcohol abusers. The flushing reaction, which does not appear to be associated with raised systemic levels of acetaldehyde, is milder than in the Oriental subjects, but is also protective against alcohol abuse. There is tentative evidence, however, that the heterozygotes, i.e. subjects with only one affected gene, show increased susceptibility to alcohol dependence, consistent with animal studies showing a dose-dependent reinforcing of alcohol consumption in response to acetaldehyde administration (Amit et al. 1980).

These studies indicate how major changes in the activity of acetaldehyde dehydrogenase(s), either genetic or acquired (e.g., drug-related inhibitions), are associated with aversive responses to alcohol consumption. Perhaps more subtle changes in enzyme activities may be reinforcing to enhanced alcohol ingestion.

Other genetic influences may be involved in the abuse and/or toxicity of alcohol. Attempts to correlate severity of alcoholic liver disease with drug-metabolizing abilities have so far not proved positive (Lanthier et al. 1984). The differing susceptibility to alcohol toxicity of women compared to men is of interest, and, again, differences in alcohol metabolism, particularly acetaldehyde accumulation, have been implicated in the greater susceptibility to liver damage in females. The basis for this gender difference is uncertain,

TABLE 9.3 Survival in alcoholic liver disease

Ethnic group	Survival (months)
Afro-Caribbeans	80
Caucasians	30
Hispanics	25
American-Indians	8

Fifty per cent median survival times for males with alcoholic liver disease. Values calculated from the data of Mendenhall et al. (1989).

but females show higher blood alcohol levels and, possibly, higher tissue acetaldehyde levels (Arthur et al. 1984; Coleharding and Wilson 1987; Loft et al. 1987; Pikkar et al. 1988) after a standard test dose of ethanol, compared to male subjects. The biochemical basis for these observations are, however, uncertain at present, but recent reports have implicated reduced metabolism of alcohol by the stomach in the enhanced female susceptibility (Frezza et al. 1990). Other suggestions include small liver volumes, enhanced metabolic clearance and altered tissue distributions in the increased susceptibility to alcohol abuse.

The Oriental flushers are protected against alcohol abuse, but certain ethnic groups appear to be more susceptible. A careful study of the prognosis of patients with severe alcoholic liver disease show striking variation in survival between different ethnic groups in the US (Table 9.3). Clearly, many factors will influence the outcome of patients admitted for treatment of alcoholic liver disease, but a biological component is likely. This is reinforced by a recent study from West London which shows that Asian–Indian immigrants appear to be more susceptible to the damaging effects of alcohol, both in terms of amount and duration of abuse (Clarke et al. 1990). The basis of this ethnic variation is uncertain; cultural factors are clearly important but genetic factors are also likely to be involved. The new approaches now available with techniques of molecular biology will considerably assist these studies. Possible genetic variants in alcohol and acetaldehyde metabolizing enzymes, in certain neurotransmitters and their receptors and in biogenic amine synthesis and metabolism, may be reflected in specific deletions or mutations which are demonstrable on examination of leucocyte DNA. Thus, a recent report has claimed that the D2 dopamine gene (A1) is significantly associated with alcoholism, compared with control subjects (Blum et al. 1990). These gene variants may, in combination with environmental, cultural or other acquired factors, predispose or prevent alcohol abuse and toxicity. This approach is likely to overcome the difficulties with the present biochemical and pharmacological methods which frequently lead to difficulties in distinguishing primary and secondary events.

TISSUE SUSCEPTIBILITY

Although the onset of alcohol abuse is attributable to a complex interaction of genetic, cultural, and biological factors, there is still a wide variation in the severity and extent of end organ damage. In particular, there is a remarkable variation in susceptibility to tissue damage, as referred to above. An important feature is that organ damage is not part of a general toxicity, but appears to show selectivity. Thus, there is clear evidence that females are more susceptible to hepatic damage, possibly related to their greater susceptibility to liver damage in general (Saunders and Williams 1983). In contrast, alcoholic heart disease is a very rare complication of chronic alcohol abuse in women (P. J. Richardson, personal communication).

To illustrate further the idiosyncratic susceptibility to selective organ damage, chronic alcoholic skeletal muscle damage will be used as a paradigm. This form of muscle damage has only relatively recently been described in detail. It is a frequent complication, affecting between one-half and two-thirds of all chronic alcohol abusers (Peters *et al.* 1985; Urbano-Marquez *et al.* 1989). Histologically, it is a Type II (anaerobic, glycolytic, fast twitch) fibre atrophy affecting proximal muscles of the pectoral and pelvic girdles. The myopathy is reversible, both clinically and histologically, in patients abstaining for at least 3 months, and available evidence, both in man and in experimental animals (Preedy and Peters 1990), indicates that the myopathy is due to a direct toxic effect of alcohol and not a secondary effect due to hormonal, nutritional or metabolic consequences of alcohol-mediated damage to other organs, including liver, the central and peripheral nervous systems or various endocrine glands.

A key question arises as to why Type II rather than Type I muscle fibres are affected. Concerning the greater susceptibility of Type II fibre-rich muscles to alcohol toxicity, it is difficult to investigate this in man as all muscles are composed of mixtures of Type I and Type II fibres. However, in the rat, although some muscles, e.g. gastrocnemius, are of mixed fibre type, in certain muscles individual fibre types predominate. Thus, soleus contains mainly Type I muscle fibres and plantaris Type II fibres (Preedy *et al.* 1989), and it is, therefore, possible to explore the biochemical basis for the increased susceptibility of the latter muscle fibres to alcohol-mediated damage, by investigating differences in the metabolism of these two muscles.

The first area of study concerned lipid and carbohydrate metabolism, as the presence and absence of mitochondria in Type I and Type II muscle fibres, respectively, is the most striking difference between these muscles. Detailed metabolic studies could not attribute the differential susceptibility to alteration in energy metabolism (Cook *et al.* 1989). However, studies of the acute effect of ethanol on protein synthesis by Type I and Type II

TABLE 9.4 Antioxidants in rat skeletal muscles

Antioxidant (mUnits mg^{-1} protein)	Soleus (Type I)	Plantaris (Type II)
Superoxide dismutase	9.10 ± 1.82	6.73 ± 1.47
Catalase	1.8 ± 0.3	0.70 ± 0.01
Glutathione reductase	7.3 ± 1.4	2.90 ± 0.01
Glutathione peroxidase	14.2 ± 5.1	7.4 ± 3.8
Selenium (pg mg^{-1} protein)	2.93 ± 1.24	2.13 ± 0.52
α-Tocopherol (pmol mg^{-1} protein)	33.1 ± 7.3	18.3 ± 4.5

Mean ± SD values for 4–6 animals. Data from C. D. Abiaka R. J. Ward, and T. J. Peters (unpublished results).

fibre-rich muscles clearly demonstrate that the latter show a greater reduction (30 per cent) compared with the former (20 per cent) (Preedy and Peters 1988a). Similar conclusions were reached in a chronic alcohol feeding study (Preedy and Peters 1988b). This suggests that the atrophy of the Type II fibres reflects a differential inhibition of protein synthesis by ethanol in these fibres. The reason for this differential effect is not yet known, but our current hypothesis implicates enhanced free radical activity.

There is considerable evidence that alcohol ingestion, both acute and chronic, leads to enhanced formation of free radicals (Peters *et al.* 1986). Table 9.4 shows preliminary data on the activities of four enzymes implicated in the scavenging of free radical and reactive oxygen species, in Type I and Type II fibre-rich muscles. In addition, levels of tissue selenium, an essential cofactor for glutathione peroxidase and for α-tocopherol (vitamin E), the principle lipid-soluble and, therefore, membrane-associated antioxidant in mammalian cells are reported. All scavengers and antioxidants show significantly lower levels in the alcohol-susceptible Type II fibres. Clearly, further work is necessary on the effects of acute and chronic alcohol administration on the levels of the free radical scavengers and antioxidants in the various muscle types and on the levels of the free radicals and their reaction products in the various tissues and components thereof, as these observations potentially offer an approach to limiting alcohol-mediated tissue damage.

The animal studies are likely to be highly relevant to human studies and this is illustrated in Fig. 9.2. Alcoholics without myopathy show serum α-tocopherol levels mostly within the normal range, whereas all patients with histologically-proven myopathy have reduced levels of the antioxidants (Ward *et al.* 1988).

Type I mitochondrial-rich fibres generate free radicals during their normal metabolic processes and therefore require, and have acquired, significant

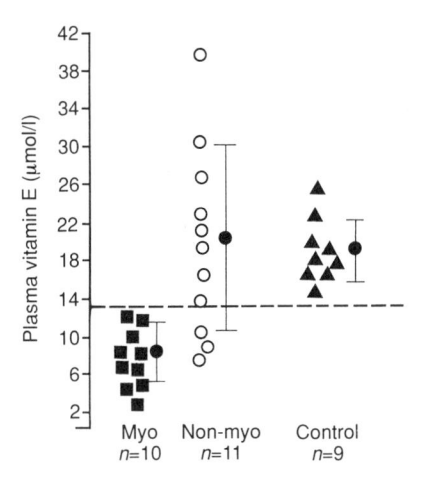

FIG. 9.2 Plasma vitamin E levels in control subjects and chronic alcohol abusers. Alcoholics are subdivided into those with (myo) or without (non-myo) histologically-proven chronic skeletal myopathy. Mean ± SD are shown for each patient group.

amounts of a wide range of antioxidant systems. Type II fibres normally generate few free radical species and on chronic exposure to ethanol are less able to neutralize these compounds formed as a consequence of ethanol metabolism. As a result, several metabolic processes, most notably protein synthesis, are inhibited. During the scavenging process α-tocopherol is degraded and thus will eventually lead to impaired antioxidant activity with further cellular damage. It is suggested that such a situation occurs in man following prolonged alcohol abuse. Whether α-tocopherol and other antioxidants will be effective in preventing alcohol-induced muscle damage is an unanswered question. Whether it is ethically justified to prescribe drugs that limit cellular damage in the face of continued alcohol abuse, when abstinence itself will lead to a reversal of the myopathy, is also controversial. Use of antioxidants in hastening recovery of abstaining alcoholics await carefully-controlled clinical trials.

CONCLUSION

Alcohol abuse occurs because of a complex interplay of genetic and environmental factors which promote or limit alcohol consumption. Individual susceptibility to abuse may relate to subtle alterations in ethanol and acetaldehyde metabolisms: individual organ susceptibility appears to relate to a complex interplay of ethanol- and acetaldehyde-mediated free radical generation and the levels and activity of cytoprotective, free radical scavengers and antioxidants. Nutritional and hormonal effects of alcoholic beverages and other toxins appear to be relatively unimportant in determining an individual's susceptibility.

ACKNOWLEDGEMENT

I am grateful to Miss Cheryl Riley for expert secretarial assistance.

REFERENCES

Amit, Z., Brown, Z. W., Rockman, G. E., Smith, B., and Amir, S. (1980). Acetaldehyde: a positive reinforcer mediating ethanol consumption. *Advances in Experimental Medicine and Biology*, **126**, 413–23.

Arthur, M. J. P., Lee, A., and Wright, R. (1984). Sex differences in the metabolism of ethanol and acetaldehyde in normal subjects. *Clinical Science*, **67**, 397–401.

Blum, K., Noble, E. P., Sheridan, P. J., Montgomery, A., Ritchie, A., Jagadeeswaran, P., Nogami, H., Briggs, A.H., and Cohen, J. (1990). Allelic association of human depamine D_2 receptor gene in alcoholism. *Journal of the American Medical Association*, **263**, 2055–60.

Clarke, M., Ahmed, N., Romaniuk, H., Marjot, D. H., and Murray-Lyon, I. M. (1990). Ethnic differences in the consequences of alcohol misuse. *Alcohol and Alcoholism*, **25**, 9–11.

Coleharding, S. and Wilson, J. R. (1987). Ethanol metabolism in men and women. *Journal of Studies on Alcohol*, **48**, 380–7.

Cook, E. B., Preedy, V. R., Peters, T. J., and Palmer, T. N. (1989). Does chronic alcohol skeletal myopathy arise secondary to impaired energy metabolism. *Alcohol and Alcoholism*, **24**, 369.

Cook, E. B., Preedy, V. R., Peters, T. J., and Palmer, T. N. (1990). Effects of chronic ethanol feeding on muscle metabolism in the rat. *Biochemical Society Transactions*, **18**, 978–9.

Ewing, J. A., Rose, B. A., and Pellizzari, E. D. (1974). Alcohol sensitivity and ethnic background. *American Journal of Psychiatry*, **131**, 206–16.

Frezza, M., DiPadova, C., Pozzato, G., Terpin, M., Baraona, E., and Lieber, C. S. (1990). High blood alcohol levels in women: role of decreased gastric alcohol dehydrogenase activity and first pass metabolism. *New England Journal of Medicine*, **322**, 95–9.

Goedde, H. W. and Agarwal, D. P. (1987). Polymorphism of aldehyde dehydrogenase and alcohol sensitivity. *Enzyme*, **37**, 29–44.

Halliwell, B. and Gutteridge, J. M. C. (1985). *Free radicals in biology and medicine*. Clarendon Press, Oxford.

Lanthier, P. L., Reshef, R., Shah, R. R., Oates, N. S., Smith, R. L., and Morgan, M. Y. (1984). Oxidation phenotyping in alcoholics with liver disease of varying severity. *Alcohol Clinical Experimental Research*, **8**, 43–441.

Loft, S., Olesen, K. L., and Dossing, M. (1987). Increased susceptibility to liver disease in relation to alcohol consumption in women. *Scandinavian Journal of Gastroenterology*, **22**, 1251.

Mendenhall, C. L. Gartside, P. S., Roselle, C. A., Grossman, C. J., Weesner, P. E., and Chedid, A. (1989). Longevity among ethnic groups with alcoholic liver disease. *Alcohol and Alcoholism*, **24**, 11–19.

Mizoi, Y., Ijiri, I., Tatsuno, Y., Kijima, T., Fujiwara, S., and Adachi, J. (1979). Relationship between facial flushing and blood acetaldehyde levels after alcohol intake. *Pharmacology, Biochemistry and Behavior*, **10**, 303–11.

Peters, T. J., Martin, F., and Ward, K. (1985). Chronic alcoholic skeletal myopathy — common and reversible. *Alcohol*, **2**, 485–9.

Peters, T. J., O'Connell, M. J., Venkatesan, S., and Ward, R. J. (1986). Evidence for free radical-mediated damage in experimental alcoholic liver disease. In C. Rice-Evans (eds), *Free radicals, cell damage and disease*, pp. 99–110. IRL Press, England.

Peters, T. J., Macpherson, A. J. S., Ward, R. J., and Yoshida, A. (1990). Acquired and genetic deficiencies of cytosolic acetaldehyde dehydrogenase. Banbury Rep No. 33, Cold Spring Harbor Laboratory, New York.

Pikkar, N. A., Wedel, M., and Hermus, R. J. J. (1988). Influence of several factors on blood alcohol concentrations after drinking alcohol. *Alcohol and Alcoholism*, **23**, 289–97.

Preedy, V. R. and Peters, T. J. (1988a). Acute effects of ethanol on protein synthesis in different muscles and muscle protein fractions of the rat. *Clinical Science*, **74**, 461–6.

Preedy, V. R. and Peters, T. J. (1988b). The effect of chronic ethanol ingestion on protein metabolism in Type I- and Type II-fibre-rich skeletal muscles of the rat. *Biochemical Journal*, **254**, 631–9.

Preedy, V. R. and Peters, T. J. (1990). Alcohol and skeletal muscle disease. *Alcohol and Alcoholism*, **25**, 177–87.

Preedy, V. R., Bateman, C. J., Salisbury, J. R., Price, A. B., and Peters, T. J. (1989). Ethanol-induced skeletal muscle myopathy. Biochemical and histochemical measurements on Type I and Type II fibre-rich muscles in the young rat. *Alcohol and Alcoholism*, **24**, 533–9.

Saunders, J. B. and Williams, R. (1983). The genetics of alcoholism: is there an inherited susceptibility to alcohol-related problems? *Alcohol and Alcoholism*, **18**, 189–217.

Shibuya, A. and Yoshida, A. (1988a). Genotypes of alcohol-metabolising enzymes in Japanese with alcohol liver disease: a strong association of the usual Caucasian-type aldehyde dehydrogenase gene (ALDH$^1_2$) with the disease. *American Journal of Human Genetics*, **43**, 744–8.

Singh, S., Fritze, G., Fang, B., Harada S., Paik, Y. K., Eckey, R., Agarwal, D. P., and Goedde, H. W. (1989). Inheritance of mitochondrial aldehyde dehydrogenase: genotyping in Chinese, Japanese and South Korean families. *Human Genetics* **83**, 119–21.

Urbano-Marquez, A., Estruch, R., Navarro-Lopez, F., Grau, J., Mont, L., and Rubin, E. (1989). The effect of alcoholism on skeletal cardiac muscle. *New England Journal of Medicine*, **320**, 409–15.

Ward, R. J., Jutla, J., Duane, P., and Peters, T. J. (1988). Reduced antioxidant status in patients with chronic alcoholic myopathy. *Biochemical Society Transactions,* **16**, 581.

Wilson J. R., McClearn F., and Johnson R. C. (1978). Ethnic variation in the use and effects of alcohol. *Drug and Alcohol Dependence,* **3**, 147–51.

Wolff, P.C. (1972). Ethnic differences in alcohol sensitivity. *Science,* **175**, 449–50.

Yoshida, A., Huang, I. Y., and Ikawa, M. (1984). Molecular abnormality of an inactive aldehyde dehydrogenase variant commonly found in Orientals. *Proceedings of the National Academy of Science,* **81**, 258–61.

Yoshida, A., Dave, V., Ward, R. J., and Peters, T. J. (1989). Cytosolic aldehyde dehydrogenase (ALDH1) variants found in alcohol flushers. *American Journal of Human Genetics,* **53**, 1–7.

10

Problem definition: the case of the benzodiazepines

MALCOLM LADER

INTRODUCTION

The concepts of abuse and addiction were found to be unsatisfactory because of problems of definition. The fashion turned to viewing this area in terms of problems, hopefully defined in operational terms of pragmatic utility. However, by no means all the difficulties of definition were solved. The case of the benzodiazepines illustrates how the definition of a problem depends on the perception of the people involved and this in turn reflects their background and outlook.

The benzodiazepines themselves achieved spectacular success, at least in commercial terms, because prescribers and patients both saw them as solving the main problems associated with their predecessors, namely, abuse, dependence, danger in overdose, and metabolic interactions with other drugs. But as this brief chapter will attempt to show, problems remained which were ignored or minimized for a long time.

THE PROBLEM OF EXTENSIVE USAGE

The benzodiazepines were perceived to be an improvement on the barbiturates mainly in terms of safety in overdose. This led to a replacement of the new for the old, plus a definite widening of usage with poorly defined indications. This was encouraged by the manufacturers as new drugs are more profitable than the old. Indeed, some of the advertising verges on the irresponsible with the 'medicalization' of normal events such as bereavement in order to justify pharmacological intervention. By 1975, the year in which benzodiazepine sales peaked in the USA, total anxiolytic and hypnotic sales accounted for about 10 per cent of all prescriptions — the benzodiazepines were the most successful drugs of all time.

Concern was expressed at the extent of usage: it was perceived as a problem in its own right (the benzodiazepine 'bonanza', Tyrer 1974) and as reflecting some underlying dependence process (the 'opium of the masses', Lader 1978). A growing chorus of opinion had urged the substitution of the barbiturates by the benzodiazepines. The so-called CURB campaign sponsored by the British Medical Association played a major role in this. Some of these people now began to question the need for this avalanche of benzodiazepine prescriptions. But whereas the disadvantages and problems associated with the barbiturates were well-known, those presumed to relate to the benzodiazepines were vague and ill-formulated. Criticisms were even at times moral rather than medical in tone. All observers agreed, however, that a major problem with the barbiturates, toxicity in overdose, was only a minor consideration with the benzodiazepines.

The moral problem was articulated by some within the medical profession but mostly by concerned lay people. For example, the Public Citizen Health Research Group in the USA wrote that, 'Prescribing valium for a situational problem is like giving a man with a broken leg morphine for his pain and telling him to keep walking' (Bargmann et al. 1982). Aldous Huxley put it thus (Brave New World Revisited, 1960).

> As things now stand, the tranquillizers may prevent some people from giving enough trouble not only to their rulers, but even to themselves. Too much tension is a disease; but so is too little. There are certain occasions when we *ought* to be tense, when an excess of tranquillity (and especially tranquillity imposed from the outside, by a chemical) is entirely inappropriate.

These criticisms are of inappropriate prescribing, the first deprecating the use of a symptomatic remedy for a deep-rooted problem, the second that the symptomatic remedy prevents the confrontation of that problem on either a personal or a societal level — 'the opium of the masses' again. The preponderance of benzodiazepine use among women has led to assertion by Women's Liberation groups that they are weapons used by male doctors to prolong the subjugation of women.

THE ADVERSE EFFECT PROBLEMS

Such unfocused allegations of problems led to a reappraisal of the properties of the benzodiazepines, starting in the late 1970s. In the increasingly unfavourable climate of perception of the benzodiazepines, what had appeared to be advantages over the more unsatisfactory barbiturates became disadvantages *vis-à-vis* non-pharmacological methods of managing anxiety and to a lesser extent, insomnia. Thus, drowsiness, fatigue, loss of coordination and decreased attention and concentration were studied in greater detail and the drawbacks of the tranquillizers became increasingly apparent. In particular, anecdotal reports of memory disturbances led to intensive evaluation of this problem using up-to-date psychological techniques (Curran 1986; Curran et al. 1987). The elderly were known to be particularly at risk, confusion and ataxia being common especially after hypnotics. One problem was subsequent falls and fractured neck of femur. Paradoxical reactions were also perceived as constituting a problem. Hostility and rage reactions occur in a small proportion of patients given a benzodiazepine, and subsequent violence can cause major problems with involvement of legal agencies.

These drug associated adverse events had been known from the early days of the usage of the tranquillizers. However, these undoubted problems had been brushed to one side in the general mood of euphoria of prescriber and patient alike, regarding the usefulness and acceptability of these drugs. Once doubts had been raised, problems were sought, found, defined and used to justify those doubts.

THE PROBLEM OF ABUSE

Abuse, the non-medical use of high doses, was assumed to be a potential problem from the start. The barbiturates and non-barbiturate successors such as meprobamate were known to be drugs of abuse, and this problem had led to the scheduling of the barbiturates on an international basis. Intravenous use carried all sorts of risks including necrosis of the extremities. Initially there was no reason to suspect that the benzodiazepines would be any different but they were not scheduled routinely. What monitoring there was, suggested that abuse was not becoming a major issue with the benzodiazepines, perhaps because of pharmacokinetic factors such as low aqueous solubility. Abuse by the oral route did however pose problems and eventually the benzodiazepines were scheduled internationally, although in many countries, a special low category of scheduling had to be instituted in order to accommodate these drugs. Sporadic outbursts of abuse involving one or other benzodiazepine were reported.

However, in the UK it became apparent that the abuse potential of the benzodiazepine was actually quite high once a suitable formulation was available. This happened with temazepam which was formulated in liquid-filled capsules to expedite absorption. Polydrug abusers charged their syringes with this liquid formulation and injected intravenously, with all the secondary problems of communication of infection such as HIV. The various manufacturers of this formulation were persuaded to reformulate either as a tablet or as a putty-like compound in the capsules. However, the abusers used great ingenuity in rendering the putty injectable by heating it or dissolving it, or the tablets, in alcohol or citric acid. Injection is not easy however and tissue damage is common.

Thus, the problem had arisen from one formulation and the belief that the benzodiazepines were not nearly as likely to be abused as their predecessors. An accident of formulation led to the true potential for abuse being realized and the problem remains. Furthermore, the newer formulations have turned the wheel back full circle, with the secondary problems of the infective and necrotic sequelae of intravenous injection being made worse by reformulating the easy-to-inject but safer liquid formulations.

THE PROBLEM OF DEPENDENCE

Two studies in the early 1960s established the potential of a benzodiazepine to induce a physical dependence state when the drug was given in high dose for weeks on end (Hollister *et al.* 1961, 1963). Thus the existence of this property of the tranquillizers was established right from the initiation of these drugs, that is, a potential problem had been identified. These studies which would now be regarded as of dubious ethicality involved artificial conditions of forced high dosage. They did not establish the likelihood of any patient starting on a therapeutic dose, escalating it up into high levels because of tolerance and dependence.

In the two decades following the introduction of the benzodiazepines, the scientific literature is punctuated with case reports of patients who had escalated their dose of tranquillizer way above the therapeutic limit. Those who had tried to discontinue the drug had suffered a withdrawal syndrome of the sedative/hypnotic type. However, little notice was taken of these reports, no problem was perceived. Indeed, despite the accrual of hundreds of such case-reports, Marks (1978) claimed that relatively few contained fully verified cases of dependence. He set these cases against the worldwide use of the benzodiazepines and concluded: 'The dependence risk with benzodiazepines is very low and is estimated to be approximately one case per 5 million patient months "at risk" for all recorded cases.'

This anodyne conclusion of no problem was based on the assumption that dependence only occurred with tolerance and escalation of dosage. This assumption was widely challenged, further information accumulated and Marks (1983) recanted.

The increasing cohort of long-term users who had not escalated their dose was seen as a problem in terms of possible adverse effects of the drugs, but also the possibility was mooted that such long-term usage reflected normal dose dependence rather than the chronicity of the underlying psychopathology. Such a possibility had been raised in the early 1970s (e.g. Covi *et al.* 1973), but dismissed as unlikely or infrequent. By the mid-

1980s the reality of such dependence had been established (e.g. Petursson and Lader 1984) and papers abounded drawing attention to this problem.

But what was the problem? Certainly, perhaps a million or more patients took a benzodiazepine chronically, many claiming therapeutic benefit. Perhaps, a third or so of these would experience problems on attempted discontinuation. But why not continue? The detailed studies of unwanted effects showed many patients to be at risk of cognitive, psychomotor, and memory disturbances but the extent of this potential problem was unknown. In some patients tolerance did seem to occur leading to symptom breakthrough and/or partial withdrawal; again extent unknown. Parallel experiments to those in problem drinkers led to questions being raised concerning neuroanatomical changes accompanied by neuropsychological deficits. But to many users, problems only seemed to arise when the medication was discontinued.

The withdrawal syndrome was an undoubted problem, often severe, sometimes prolonged and occasionally intolerable. Nevertheless, most patients who managed to withdraw and stayed drug-free described an improvement, so by inference the previous drug-taking constituted a problem. For others, the entire process of withdrawal was a major management problem involving the patient, relatives and friends, doctors, nurses etc. Belatedly, the medical profession perceived a problem and sought to limit the usage of benzodiazepines by issuing guidelines (College Statement 1989).

The public also perceived a problem. Radio and television programmes were followed by a flood of correspondence from sufferers and their relatives which was much greater than any previously publicized topics. The prescribers and the pharmaceutical industry were castigated for causing this problem by their cavalier and indiscriminate prescribing and promotion. Finally, the legal profession became involved because benzodiazepine users and ex-users perceived that they had been damaged by these drugs and sought redress from the manufacturers.

REFERENCES

Bargmann, E., Wolfe, S. M., Levin, J., and the Public Citizen Health Research Group (1982). *Stopping valium*. Public Citizen's Health Research Group, Washington.

College Statement: Royal College of Psychiatrists (1988). Benzodiazepines and dependence. *Bulletin of the Royal College of Psychiatrists*, **12**, 107–9.

Covi, L., Lipman, R. S., Pattison, J. H., Derogatis, L. R., and Uhlenhuth, E. H. (1973). Length of treatment with anxiolytic sedatives and response to their sudden withdrawal. *Acta Psychiatrica Scandinavica*, **49**, 51–64.

Curran, H. V. (1986). Tranquillising memories: a review of the effects of benzodiazepines on human memory. *Biological Psychology*, **23**, 179–213.

Curran, H. V., Schiwy, W., and Lader, M. (1987). Differential amnesic properties of benzodiazepines: a dose–response comparison of two drugs with similar elimination half-lives. *Psychopharmacology*, **92**, 358–64.

Hollister, L. E., Motzenbecker, F. P., and Degan, R. O. (1961). Withdrawal reactions from chlordiazepoxide ('Librium'). *Psychopharmacologia*, **2**, 63–8.

Hollister, L. E., Bennett, J. L., Kimbell, I., Savage, C., and Overall, J. E. (1963). Diazepam in newly admitted schizophrenics. *Diseases of the Nervous System*, **24**, 746–50.

Huxley, A. (1960). *Brave new world revisited*; p. 61. Harper & Row, New York.

Lader, M. (1978). Benzodiazepines — the opium of the masses? *Neuroscience*, **3**, 159–65.

Marks, J. (1978). *The benzodiazepines. Use, overuse, misuse, abuse*. MTP, Lancaster, UK.

Marks, J. (1983). The benzodiazepines — for good or evil. *Neuropsychobiology*, **10**, 115–26.

Petursson, H. and Lader M. (1984). *Dependence on tranquillizers*. Oxford University Press, Oxford.

Tyrer, P. (1974). The benzodiazepine bonanza. *The Lancet*, **ii**, 709–10.

11

The problems perspective: implications for prevention policies

REGINALD G. SMART*

INTRODUCTION

Whether prevention policies and programmes have a 'dependence' or a 'problems' approach will influence how activities are planned, and their content, as well as their overall aims. This chapter will attempt to show how the dimensions of a dependence- and problems-based prevention approach differ, and some details for the problems approach will be given.

In a dependence approach to prevention programmes policies focus on dependent individuals or those at high risk for dependence. In practice this means preventing dependence among those drug users who have not yet fallen prey to it, and preventing dependence from worsening among those who have. Of course, dependence has many meanings, and there is 'no clear-cut universally accepted definition of dependence' (see Babor 1990, for a review). In this chapter we will take the meaning of the medical model of dependence, as it probably is the most widely understood. It includes the concept of 'dependence (being) a distinct and progressive disease entity having physical origins or manifestations, and requiring medical treatment for proper management' (Babor 1990), and a state of physical adaptation to drugs characterized by tolerance and withdrawal symptoms, and an emotional state of craving.

Problems due to alcohol and drugs are undefined in advance and we look to the scientist or prevention programmer for a definition each time the word 'problem' is used. Problem definition involves values, attitudes, and assumptions in a way that dependence does not. Whether a particular social or psychological event is a problem depends upon the observer and the context. Many parents would define any cannabis use by an eight-year-old

---

* Addiction Research Foundation, 33 Russell Street, Toronto, Canada. The views expressed in this paper are those of the author and do not necessarily reflect those of the Addiction Research Foundation.

child as 'a problem', but they might not if it is by a college student. Religious, abstaining parents might define any alcohol use by adolescents as a problem.

There are drug related problems about which there will be near total agreement, e.g. drug related traffic accidents, falls, drownings, and all the physical sequelae of heavy alcohol and drug use such as liver cirrhosis, 'crack' lung, hepatitis, or HIV infection. There are also social or familial consequences which will usually be called 'problems', e.g. marital breakdown, family violence, or job loss, but there is room to disagree. However, some problems defined by society or parents are enjoyed and sought after by the user, e.g. intoxication or being arrested or warned by the police. Adolescent heavy drinkers often set out to get drunk on weekends and are disappointed if they do not. In some delinquent groups it is worth bragging about if your drinking attracts the attention of police.

LEVELS OF PROBLEMS AND DEPENDENCE

We can see from Colin Drummond's chapter that almost all dependent persons have social and physical problems from their drug use. However, many people with such problems are not dependent on any drug. The differences in numbers of dependent people and those with alcohol and drug problems can be very striking. For example, in a recent survey about 9 per cent of adults in Ontario scored two or more on the CAGE scale for alcohol problems (Smart and Adlaf 1989). This is the level usually associated with serious problems in need of attention. This amounts to about 585 000 adults out of a population of 6.5 million. If we include all persons admitting any sort of alcohol problem on the CAGE, the number is more than a million. However, the Jellinek Estimation Formula gives about 180 000 alcoholics in Ontario in 1989, or only 31 per cent of those with a serious alcohol problem, and 20 per cent of those with some problem.

The same differences between levels of problems and probable dependence can be seen for young people. Only 0.9 per cent of students aged about 12–18 in Ontario had ever seen a doctor or been to a hospital for a drinking problem, which might be taken as evidence of dependence (Smart and Adlaf 1989). However, 5.8 per cent had been arrested or warned by police for drinking and 4.8 per cent wished they could drink less. We could assume that those students with alcohol problems are five or six times as numerous as those with a dependency on alcohol.

A problem approach to prevention must deal with the large numbers of potential and actual victims. However, a focus on dependent individuals can involve relatively few people in the population with many similar characteristics. If 20 per cent–25 per cent of the adult population has an alcohol or drug problem of some magnitude, the prevention task is enormous. It suggests the need for a wide range of efforts, including specialized programmes, mass media involvement, and efforts by professionals at every level. It also suggests that targets should be set in terms of the problems to be defined as worthy of prevention. Of course, good programmes will select a few serious alcohol or drug problems for special attention, e.g. drinking–driving; alcohol related violence, etc. A major task for policy makers is, then, to define drug and alcohol problems, and select those most deserving of special attention.

TARGET GROUPS FOR PREVENTION

Dependency and problem based programmes would be very different in their focus on young people, especially for alcohol. For example, rates of hospital separations for alcohol dependence in Canada are about 70 per 100 000 for the age group 45–64, but only 21 per 100 000 for the 20–24 category (Adrian 1988). However, in our recent surveys the 20–24 age group contains the largest proportions of those with alcohol problems on the CAGE, and the largest number of people drinking five or more drinks on a single occasion (Adlaf and Smart 1989). Also, the 20–24 age group has the highest rate of accident rates involving alcohol, a rate far larger than the 45–64 group (74 per 100 000 vs 13 per 100 000).

The differences are even greater if we consider liver cirrhosis as an indicator of alcohol dependence. Rates are highest among those aged 65–74 (89.8 per 100 000) and almost non-existent among those aged less than 24 (about 2.0 per 100 000) (Adrian 1988). A dependency based prevention programme should focus mainly on the middle aged and the older age groups. However, a problem based prevention programme should focus on students and young adults, but not necessarily to the exclusion of older persons.

A somewhat similar situation occurs with gender. Rates of hospital separations for alcohol dependence are more than three times as high for males as females, but the ratio of males to females reporting drinking five or more drinks on an occasion is much closer (68 per cent vs 40 per cent females) (Adrian 1988). Also, the ratio of males and females reporting drinking and driving is closer (58.2 per cent vs 32.8 per cent) in at least one Canadian survey (Transport Canada 1984). Probably alcohol prevention requires some male focus but not exclusively if a wide range of problems are considered.

Problem prevention programmes involving drugs other than alcohol also require some orientation towards youth and young adults. People receiving treatment for drug dependence in Canada have a median age of about 27

(Adrian 1988). Our study of cocaine users indicated that most had been using cocaine for about seven years before serious problems developed (Erickson *et al.* 1987). However, surveys indicate that rates of most illicit drugs are highest among those of high school age (13–18). Typically, surveys show that students are much more likely than adults in general to use cocaine and cannabis. Ages at first use, for drugs such as cannabis and cocaine are about 15 and 16. If prevention programmes are to be effective, they should be instituted before the first decisions are made to use drugs.

THE PROBLEM PREVENTION FOCUS

The problem prevention approach will focus on what might be called 'single event' problems. Whereas dependence on alcohol and drugs typically develops slowly and may take years to achieve, serious alcohol and drug problems can arise from use on a single occasion. Some reports of strokes and deaths from cocaine have indicated that they occurred on the first use of cocaine and without any other concomitant drug use (Smart and Anglin 1987; Smart 1991). Traffic accidents are another example and only 40 per cent of drivers in alcohol-related accidents (Vingilis 1983) are alcoholics. Some others are problem drinkers, but many are normal drinkers. Single event drinking can also lead to alcohol-related drownings, boating accidents, snowmobile accidents, and fires.

We have argued earlier that the problem approach argues for a 'youthful focus'. Most youthful drinking is heavy drinking on a single occasion, usually a planned weekend party. About 35 per cent of students in our survey (Smart and Adlaf 1989) had been drunk in the past four weeks (5 per cent, four or more times), however, less than 1 per cent are daily drinkers and even fewer would be 'dependent'. A problem focus in the prevention of drug-related accidents is also required as poisonings most often occur among young children, not those who are dependent (Adrian 1988).

Any problem focus in prevention must take account of deaths and injuries related to the use of alcohol and drugs in heavier than usual amounts. In the case of drugs with rapid effects, such as cocaine, doses normal for heavy users can result in serious accidents for non-tolerant users. The message of the 1970s, 'Speed Kills', was usually interpreted as referring to a long term consequence, but those who created the message were also warning about its acute effects. Many prevention programmes for alcohol problems are not designed to affect dependency rates but are problem centred, e.g. avoiding drinking-driving, intoxication, or arrests for drug use.

TOBACCO AND ALCOHOL IN THE PROBLEM APPROACH TO PREVENTION

The extent to which different problem based prevention approaches can be applied to different drugs or substances is rarely considered. Usually, different control policies and educational campaigns are developed for the three types of drugs. Of course these approaches must take account of the legal nature of alcohol and tobacco, and their wide availability.

A 'problem' approach for tobacco is probably inappropriate. Social or 'non-dependent' smoking is not very common. Among students in Ontario 46 per cent of smokers smoked every day (Smart and Adlaf 1989). However, among adults almost 90 per cent of smokers were daily smokers (Adrian 1988), and presumably they are dependent smokers.

Tobacco has a very high dependence potential, and little recreational use. This means that smoking in all its forms can be the target of smoking prevention programmes. Of course, with alcohol and cannabis, the large number of social drinkers and cannabis users militates against that approach. With smoking, complete eradication of the product can be the aim. More effective controls can be introduced, e.g. very high prices can be charged, advertising can be banned and smokers can be excluded from public places.

More than with other drugs, primary prevention of smoking means preventing dependence. Prevention programmes discourage smoking in any form rather than encourage 'safe' smoking or minimal levels, as is done with alcohol. In this sense smoking prevention is similar to prevention of illicit drug use. Because of illegality, cannabis and cocaine have no widely accepted social and legal use, although they do in certain segments of society. Illegal drug use is always 'a problem', and prevention for illegal drugs can include arguments against any sort of use (e.g. you might get caught). Usually tobacco and illegal drugs are seen as 'bad' substances and fair game for any kind of government control.

Alcohol prevention approaches are the most difficult to get right as alcohol is accepted and liked by much of the world. Safe levels of drinking such as no more than four drinks, three times a week have been suggested (Sanchez-Craig 1986). Safe levels of tobacco smoking and cannabis use may be suggested but will not have a wide acceptability among health specialists.

Many drinkers of alcohol have no problems. Infrequent users of illicit drugs may have no physical or psychological problems, but there is the ever present risk of apprehension by police. Also, the large number of alcohol users without problems creates a constituency which argues for, or tolerates, a weak level of alcohol control on availability. Efforts to raise the prices of alcoholic beverages substantially for preventive means (Brunn *et al.* 1975) are likely to create a negative reaction among drinkers and politicians. However, those opposed to price controls on tobacco consumption are a much smaller and weaker constituency.

A DEPENDENCE BASED APPROACH TO PREVENTION

If we take dependence to be a state of physical adaptation involving tolerance, withdrawal symptoms, and craving then only the heaviest users of alcohol and drugs (except tobacco) are included. We know that alcoholics in treatment consume an average of 12–15 drinks per day, a very high level of consumption. Colin Drummond found that dependence and problems are correlated in a hospitalized sample, as are dependence and consumption. However, problems and consumption are not correlated. Dependent drinkers are very heavy consumers and also have personal, physical, and financial problems. Prevention of dependence then is likely to involve the prevention of many serious social problems and heavy consumption as well. Prevention of alcohol problems other than dependency will involve less emphasis on heavy, long term consumption.

Prevention of dependence with its physical dimensions, suggests approaches which focus on the heaviest users, e.g. alcoholics, heroin addicts, daily cannabis users, etc. Some have suggested that it could also involve a genetics or eugenics approach, but such efforts are likely to be unacceptable and we do not consider that here.

The prevention of alcoholism (alcohol dependence) has been attempted with physician based programmes and they show promise. Physicians often fail to make the correct diagnosis of alcoholism in up to 90 per cent of their patients (Saunders 1990). Several efforts have been made to improve the existing alcoholism screening devices available to physicians (see Saunders, 1990 for a review). Cyr and Wartman (1988) used the MAST with patients in an ambulatory medical clinic and found that 20 per cent received a score indicating alcoholism. Surprisingly, the best questions were not 'how much do you drink' but 'have you ever had a drinking problem' and 'when was your last drink'.

Several approaches to get physicians involved in secondary prevention have been successful. Heather *et al.* (1987) have been successful with a DRAMS approach (drinking sensibly and moderately with self-control), which uses instruction for the physician, monitoring of the number of drinks taken by the patient, blood tests, and a self-help manual for patients. A simple but effective approach in Malmo, Sweden, has been to provide heavy drinkers with data on their liver enzyme levels (Kristenson and Hood 1984). Secondary prevention of alcohol dependence on a large scale requires the involvement of physicians, and the utilization of existing technologies.

Attempting the same approach with illegal drug abuse may be much more difficult but is worth a few trials. Cannabis and cocaine users are often younger than heavy drinkers (average 36.4 years in Heather's study). Unfortunately, young people visit their physicians less often and hence are less accessible to their influence. Also, the self-help manuals and body fluid tests for drug-related physical problems are not so readily available.

A further approach to secondary prevention of alcoholism is to increase the numbers of alcoholics going into treatment. Several countries have found declines in liver cirrhosis deaths and hospital admissions for alcohol dependency. For example, Smart and Mann (1987) found that liver cirrhosis rates had declined in Ontario by 28 per cent between 1974 and 1983, and other indicators fell by larger amounts, although per capita consumption declined by only 3 per cent. During that time, rates of admission of alcoholics to treatment almost doubled in Ontario as the treatment network was greatly expanded. Decreased hospital separations for liver cirrhosis were associated with increased levels of treatment across Ontario (Mann *et al.* 1988). Later research has also shown that increases in membership in Alcoholics Anonymous in the US are associated with decreased liver cirrhosis deaths. A major secondary prevention effort should involve creating more treatment services and self-help programmes for alcoholics. In many countries such services are still expensive, or inaccessible to alcoholics, or unacceptable in some other way. Increasing treatment levels should also reduce the indicators of drug dependency but research on this has not yet been done.

SUGGESTIONS FOR PROBLEM BASED PREVENTION PROGRAMMES

There is no doubt that establishing an effective primary prevention programme for alcohol and drug problems is a formidable task. We can see the outline of such programmes but far more research is needed before a final programme can be recommended. Any problem based approach must include the prevention of dependency along the lines suggested, as dependency is a major problem. Also, a problem based approach must be focused on large segments of the population, and hence be expensive and large in scope and intensity. The approach must focus on young people (but not exclusively) and recognize that women also have alcohol and drug problems. There is also a need to prevent a wide variety of problems from both 'single event' and long term consequences of drug use.

All national prevention programmes must allocate time and resources to supply and demand reduction in the best possible way. Demand reduction efforts include education programmes, mass media information efforts, and secondary prevention. Supply reduction involves controls on price and availability, and penalties for illegal possession and trafficking. Most national anti-drug programmes as well as the international effort, seem focused on supply reduction. With regard to alcohol and tobacco the situation is quite different. Controls on alcohol and tobacco availability seem weak, at least compared to those for illicit drugs, and educational efforts are typically preferred.

Some recent research has been done on the effectiveness of supply reduction strategies, especially those employed by the USA. The war on drugs, especially cocaine, of the past few years has included greater customs and coastguard activities, increased arrest levels for users and dealers, and confiscation of drug profits. Despite the cost and size of the effort the results must be seen as disappointing, as cocaine price levels have largely been unaffected and the number of heavy users has shown little decline (Nadelmann 1989). This has brought calls for a cessation of controls and 'legalization' of cocaine. However, it is difficult to estimate what the increase in number of cocaine users and cocaine dependent persons would be under any system of 'legalization'. Without an assurance that these levels would be low, many will not accept an end to supply controls.

Experience with ending controls on alcohol after Prohibition suggests that drug problems would increase substantially after controls were lifted, and therefore a cautious approach is suggested. The effectiveness of controls on alcohol availability through price, hours of sale, and the like is well accepted (Bruun *et al.* 1975) but the effectiveness of similar controls on drugs is often doubted. Probably, all prevention efforts require controls on the availability of drugs liable to cause dependency. The task of policy makers is to make controls effective while having a minimal negative impact on users through criminalization.

The demand reduction approach has attracted more research than has supply reduction. Many studies of school- and community-based programmes have been made. In general, school-based alcohol and drug education programmes have the desired positive impacts on attitudes and knowledge levels (Moskowitz 1989), but relatively weak and inconsistent impacts on behaviours such as drinking and drug use. An analysis of 127 such programmes showed that the most effective programmes are of longer duration (Schaps *et al.* 1981), but most drug education programmes are too short to have much impact. In Ontario, for example, students get only one or two classes per year on alcohol and about the same number on drugs. An interesting meta-analysis of 143 alcohol and drug education programmes showed that peer based or refusal skills programmes (e.g. 'Just Say No') for alcohol, drugs, and tobacco had the largest positive effects for students in general (Tobler 1986). However, didactic programmes based on increasing knowledge levels were largely ineffective. Alternative programmes, e.g. supplying after-school activities; recreational pursuits, were most effective for high risk students such as drug users, delinquents, and problem students. These results clearly show that the type and duration of the programme matter, and that programmes must be tailored to the characteristics of the students involved.

In the past few years prevention programmes have taken on a broader focus in the community as a whole. The Stanford Heart Disease Prevention Project (Farquhar *et al.* 1977) has been the model for many of these programmes. It emphasized a broad approach with mass media programmes, special efforts to get high risk people to change their diets and smoking, and to change levels of awareness. Several community action programmes on alcohol related problems have been reported (e.g. Casswell and Gilmore 1989) with positive effects. Also some community based programmes for adolescent drug abuse have been effective. Pentz *et al.* (1989) described a programme including mass media, a school based programme for youth, parent education, and community action and policy components. It had a positive impact on alcohol and cigarette consumption as well as cannabis use. These community based programmes will be the basis of many future prevention efforts, despite their size and relatively high cost.

The last prevention concept to be discussed is 'health promotion'. It means supporting or helping 'people in their efforts to gain, regain or sustain levels of physical, emotional, social and spiritual health that are sufficient for them to function well in society' (Shain and Hershfield 1991). The theory is that if personal resources can be strengthened, then alcohol and drug problems are less likely to develop. Typically, the health promotion approach is not directed at the elimination or prevention of problems or dependence, but at the development of personal strength which will avoid problems in the future. Of course, the broadest health promotion approach encompasses the specific prevention efforts we have described. However, health promotion also includes positive efforts to increase health through better fitness, diet, lifestyle changes, stress management, and improved use of leisure time. It is too early to be sure what the ultimate effects of health promotion activities will be on alcohol and drug problems, as such programmes take a long time to achieve their aims. Health promotion concepts will guide the development of many primary prevention efforts in the near future and should receive the attention of researchers.

SOME CONCLUSIONS

Prevention based on a problems model would emphasize approaches directed to youth and women as well as men, and pay attention to 'single event' problems. If we seek to prevent only dependence we ignore many of the common drug problems. Of course, the scale of problem prevention efforts must be much greater and include those specifically for dependence. Prevention efforts must include controls on availability and carefully tailored, and intensive educational programmes. At present, the most promising approaches seem to involve multi-factor community programmes, and those intensive programmes tailored to the needs of a specific group. However, primary and secondary prevention should be seen as research fields and not ones where final pronouncement can be made.

REFERENCES

Adlaf, E. M. and Smart, R. G. (1989). *The Ontario adult alcohol and other drug use survey 1977–1989*. Addiction Research Foundation, Toronto.

Adrian, M. (1988). *Statistics on alcohol and drug use in Canada and other countries*, Vols I and II. Addiction Research Foundation, Toronto.

Babor, T. F. (1990). Social, scientific and medical issues in the definition of alcohol dependence. In Edwards, G. and Lader, M. (eds) *The nature of drug dependence*, pp. 19–40. Oxford University Press.

Bruun, K., Edwards G., Lumio, M., Mäkelä, K., Pan, L., Popham, R. E. *et al.* (1975). *Alcohol control policies in public health perspective*. Finnish Foundation for Alcohol Studies, Helsinki.

Casswell, S. and Gilmore, L. (1989). An evaluated community action project on alcohol. *Journal of Studies on Alcohol*, **50**, 339–46.

Cyr, M. G. and Wartman, S. A. (1988). The effectiveness of routine screening questions in the detection of alcoholism. *Journal of the American Medical Association*, **259**, 51–4.

Erickson, P. G., Adlaf, E. M. Murray, G. F., and Smart, R. G. (1987). *The steel drug: cocaine in perspective*. D. C. Heath, Lexington, Massachusetts.

Farquhar, J. W., Maccaby, N., Wood, P. D., Alexander, J. K., Breitrose, H., Brown, B. W. *et al.* (1977). Community education for vascular health. *Lancet*, **i**, 1192–5.

Heather, N., Campion, P. D., Neville, R. G., and Maccabe, D. (1987). Evaluation of a controlled drinking minimal intervention for problem drinkers in general practice (the DRAMS scheme). *Journal of the Royal College of General Practitioners*, **37**, 358–63.

Kristenson, H. and Hood, H. (1984). The impact of alcohol on health in the general population: a review with particular reference to experience in Malmo. *British Journal of Addiction*, **79**, 139–45.

Mann, R. E., Smart, R.G., Anglin, L., and Rush, B. R. (1988). Are decreases in liver cirrhosis rates a result of increased treatment for alcoholism? *British Journal of Addiction*, **83**, 683–8.

Moskowitz, J. M. (1989). The primary prevention of alcohol problems: a critical review of the research literature. *Journal of Studies on Alcohol*, **50**, 54–88.

Nadelmann, E. A. (1989). Drug prohibition in the United States: costs, consequences and alternatives. *Science*, **245**, 939–47.

Pentz, M. A., Dwyer, J. H., MacKinnon, D. P., Flay, B. R., Hansen, W. B., Wang, E. Y. *et al.* (1989). A multi community trial for primary abuse of adolescent drug abuse. *Journal of the American Medical Association*, **261**, 3259–66.

Sanchez-Craig, M. (1986). How much is too much? Estimates of hazardous drinking based on client's self reports. *British Journal of Addiction*, **81**, 251–6.

Saunders, J. B. (1990). Early identification of alcohol problems. *Canadian Medical Association Journal*, **143**, 1060–9.

Schaps, E., Di Bartolo, R., Moskowitz, J., Palley, C. S., and Churgin, S. (1981). A review of 127 drug abuse prevention program evaluations. *Journal of Drug Issues*, **11**, 17–43.

Shain, M. and Hershfield, L. (1991). *The abuse and misuse of other drugs: prevention through health promotion.* Addiction Research Foundation, Toronto.

Smart, R. G. (1991). Crack cocaine use: a review of prevalence and adverse effects. *American Journal of Alcohol Abuse*, **17**, 13–26.

Smart, R. G. and Adlaf, E. M. (1989). *The Ontario student drug use survey: trends between 1977–1989.* Addiction Research Foundation, Toronto.

Smart, R. G. and Anglin, L. (1987). Do we know the lethal dose of cocaine? *Journal of Forensic Sciences*, **32**, 303–12.

Smart, R. G. and Mann, R. E. (1987). Large decreases in alcohol-related problems following a slight reduction in alcohol consumption in Ontario, 1975–1983. *British Journal of Addiction*, **82**, 285–91.

Tobler, N. S. (1986). Meta analysis of 143 adolescent drug prevention programs. *Journal of Drug Issues*, **16**, 537–67.

Transport Canada (1984). *A national household survey on drinking and driving: knowledge, attitudes and behaviours of Canadian drivers.* Transport Canada, Ottawa.

Vingilis, E. (1983). Drinking drivers and alcoholics: are they from the same population? In Smart, R. G., Glaser, F. B., Israel, Y., Kalant, H., Popham, R. E., and Schmidt, W. (eds), *Research advances in alcohol and drug problems*, Vol. 7 Plenum, New York.

12

Treatment strategies within a problems framework

D. COLIN DRUMMOND

INTRODUCTION

Other chapters in this volume have charted the rise of the problems concept. The principal way in which this concept differs from earlier addiction concepts is in the focus of concern. An addiction perspective focuses on the underlying causes which may bring about a variety of problematic consequences. Examples of such causes include variously, a disease process, personality disorder, mental illness, social disadvantage, moral torpitude, or genetic disorder. Social, psychological, or physical consequences, including withdrawal and other dependence phenomena, are seen as symptoms of the underlying disorder (Jellinek 1960). The individual suffering from the disorder is a captive of the natural history process, the symptoms displaying at various times progression and regression (Jellinek 1952). This can be described as a 'constellation model' of substance-related problems: problems, dependence, and abnormal drug consummatory behaviour represent a group of related phenomena which, when found together, reflect the existence of the underlying abnormal, disordered, or diseased state. Individuals displaying such a constellation of symptoms are qualitatively different from the rest of the drug taking population, in addition to simply consuming more of the drug than their 'non-addicted' counterparts.

The problems perspective on the other hand, emphasizes that various consequences or disabilities of substance use are of important concern in their own right. Within such a view, dependence phenomena are regarded simply as further problematic consequences of heavy substance use, and as having no causal significance in the development of problems. The concept of impaired control over drug intake, important to addiction theories, does not feature within the problems framework (Fingarette 1988). (It should be noted, however, that some descriptions of the problems perspective are not so different from an addiction perspective in that alternative causal explanations are put forward (Gorman 1989.) A problems perspective can, therefore, be described as a 'disaggregation model' of substance-related problems. Increased substance use results in an increased severity and frequency of occurrence of both problems and dependence (decreased use resulting in the opposite), but the consequences bear no causal relationship to either consumption of the substance or to each other.

Within a problems perspective then, concern is focused on such problems, for example, as the threat posed to society and the individual by HIV infection or hepatic cirrhosis rather than on heroin addiction or alcoholism per se. The question of whether the individual affected by the problems is addicted to or dependent on the substance, or indeed why the substance is being taken in a particular way (e.g. by injection as opposed to orally), are not of importance within such a framework.

Based on these two different theoretical frameworks, rival and diametrically opposed treatment strategies aimed at alleviating problems related to substance use already exist. Which way should treatment services develop: towards an addiction-focused or a problems-focused approach? The aim of this chapter is to explore the implications of these two theoretical perspectives for treatment services, and to attempt to find a *rapprochement* between the opposing factions. First, however, it is necessary to explore the competing philosophies which might underlie the problems and addiction perspectives.

RIVAL PHILOSOPHIES

Palliation vs cure

In medical terminology, the champion of the addiction perspective might see the problems framework as lacking; as treatment of the symptoms rather than the illness, or indeed, as palliation rather than cure. Undoubtedly, these are value laden terms, subject to a variety of interpretations and therefore open to dismissal as over-simplistic and 'medicocentric'. Nevertheless, it is important to remember that the majority of health care personnel, in the field of alcoholism (at least in the western world), are engaged in the treatment of addiction with the implicit goal of cure. The debate as to whether alcoholism is or is not a disease remains a heated one (Fingarette 1988; Gorman 1989; *Independent* 1990), as indeed does the debate surrounding the question of whether the term 'alcoholism' should be retained or tossed onto the scrap heap (*British Journal of Addiction* 1987). To suggest that there may be no completely effective treatment for alcoholism, or that the alcoholic should contemplate a goal which falls short of complete abstinence, amounts in many circles to heresy. Other, perhaps less dogmatic treatment personnel, may on occasion accept that a definitive cure for

Treatment strategies within a problems framework 181

alcoholism has not yet been found, but continue to live in hope that one day this will come to pass. To this group, any approach which does not address the phenomenon of addiction is doomed to failure. In denouncing the efforts of the 'priesthood' and the 'moralist', for example, Trotter (1804) observed:

> Both have meant well.... But the physical influence of custom, confirmed into habit, interwoven with the actions of our sentient system, and reacting to our mental part have been entirely forgotten. The perfect knowledge of those remote causes which first induced the propensity to vinous liquors, whether they sprung from situation in life, or depended on any particular temperament of body, is necessary for conducting the cure.

Although something of a moralist himself, his attack was aimed more at formulations which did not recognize the importance of the impairment of will-power aspect of drunkenness (as well as, of course, claiming ownership of the field for the 'discerning physician'). Trotter might well have levelled the same criticism at contemporary purveyors of a problems perspective: dismissing their failure to address the important issues as he saw them, and merely aiming at palliation. But does a problems framework imply palliation, and if so, should such an aim be dismissed? Clearly the issues are much more complex than this simple dichotomy.

Figure 12.1 shows a variety of contemporary treatment approaches, superimposed on a dimension which ranges from those which are principally problem focused to those which are principally addiction focused. It is important to note that the approaches do not occupy fixed positions on this dimension and that in practice, they may be implemented differently by individual agencies or practitioners. Certain approaches, however, can best be seen as exclusively palliative: those which aim to alleviate only the consequences of substance use, without attempting to alter the underlying mode of substance use or the addictive behaviour. The prescribing of certain pharmacological agents to relieve physical or mental illness caused by substance use, where no attempt is made to deal with the drug use itself, clearly fall into this category (e.g. antidepressants to relieve alcohol-related depressive symptoms, histamine antagonists to treat alcohol-related peptic ulcers, laxatives for opiate-induced constipation). Surgical procedures such as liver transplantation for sufferers of advanced alcoholic liver disease, and coronary artery bypass surgery for individuals with smoking-related coronary artery disease represent further examples. Rehousing or supportive psychotherapy, when conducted in the absence of advice or assistance to the individual to cut down or abstain from drug use, might conceivably help to make the individual's life more bearable, but are likely to have only a minimal and temporary impact. In many cases, however, certain approaches which might be seen as palliative can reduce harm caused by

FIG. 12.1 *Problem focused and addiction focused approaches.*

	Harm reduction		
	Palliative.	**Change-orientated**	**Curative**
Pharmacological	Symptomatic treatments e.g. antidepressants H_2 antagonists	Drug substitution e.g. methadone nicotine gum	Opiate antagonists 'Craving' inhibitors
Psychological	Supportive psychotherapy	Self control strategies e.g. self-help manuals brief cognitive behaviour therapy cue exposure	Insight-orientated psychotherapy Aversion therapy
Social	Social support e.g. rehousing job finding	Public education campaigns Legislative controls e.g. taxation licencing	Punishment Social reform
Miscellaneous	Surgical e.g. liver transplant	Sterile injecting equipment	Spiritual reawakening Moral reform

Problem focused ←--→ Addiction focused drugs, and may even be life-saving. Withholding them on the condition of a change in the individual's drug taking behaviour could be seen as unethical.

In comparison, treatment approaches aimed at cure (or at least, lasting recovery) have a tremendous allure within the caring professions, partly for reasons of professional training. The owner of the definitive cure for addiction can also enjoy power through professional hegemony, as well as potentially considerable financial gain (Miller and Hester 1986a). In addition to the possible personal motives of the professional, there is pressure on treatment personnel from society to find a 'quick fix', a technological solution, to what represents a sizeable and costly social problem. While it is currently unfashionable to profess the possession of a cure, except perhaps in parts (although by no means all) of the private sector, there are a number of treatments which aim to make an impact on the addiction rather than the related problems. Many, such as psychosurgery and aversion therapy, have fallen into disuse, while others are still commonly practised.

Several drugs aimed at inhibiting or blocking 'craving' for alcohol, cocaine or heroin are under development, and some are prescribed to clinical populations. Opiate antagonists such as naltrexone, which block the reinforcing effects of this class of drugs, also currently enjoy some popularity (Kleber 1985; Brewer *et al.* 1988). Alcohol antagonists are still at the development stage. Electroacupuncture for opiate and alcohol dependence has its champions (Patterson, 1986), although the majority of the treatment system awaits convincing scientific evidence to support claims of effectiveness. The acquisition of insight into one's addiction through intensive psychotherapy has for many years been a mainstay of specialized treatment for addiction (Emrick 1975). Although now seldom used, aversion therapy had at one time a sizeable following of supporters. In several countries, punishment through imprisonment has been used as a method of 'treatment' of drug addiction, again aiming to cure what is believed to be the underlying cause. Still other approaches rely on the development of spiritual rebirth as a means of overcoming the addiction.

Pragmatism vs purism

There are several treatment approaches, including some of those illustrated in Figure 12.1, which fall some way short of attempting to cure the addiction without amounting to mere palliation. These are located in the central part of the figure, and have been labelled 'change-orientated harm reduction' approaches. They all share the common aim of attempting to reduce harm through effecting some change in either the amount or the mode of substance use, without necessarily attempting to impact upon the addiction itself. Some can be regarded as essentially pragmatic approaches in that the existence of the underlying dependence and its influence on drug taking behaviour are not in dispute, but that other, principally public health objectives such as preventing the spread of HIV infection, are of higher priority than attempting to alter the addictive process itself. Examples of this include drug substitution with oral methadone or nicotine chewing gum, the encouragement of less risky behaviour through the provision of bleach, sterile injecting equipment, and advice on safer injecting practices.

Recent descriptions of such harm reduction approaches emphasize the concept of a hierarchy of goals, namely that while lasting abstinence or recovery from the addiction represent ultimate, longer-term goals in treatment, more pragmatic intermediate goals may be more quickly and easily achieved in the short term (ACMD 1988). Further, not all drug takers will be willing to commit themselves to higher goals which may be more difficult to achieve.

While such problem focused approaches have gained a wide degree of acceptance in the treatment community in Europe and parts of the US (although the provision of sterile injecting equipment remains illegal in most parts of the US), many helping agencies including some self-help organizations regard such intermediate goals which fall short of complete abstinence, as unacceptable. Similarly, there is considerable resistance, in many parts of the alcoholism treatment community to a controlled drinking goal (in a sense, the alcoholism equivalent of harm reduction). On occasion this has reached the point of vitriolic attacks on those who disagree with the total abstinence dictum (Maltzman 1989).

Optimism vs pessimism

Some approaches in Figure 12.1 can be seen as differing in the degree of optimism concerning the ability of the individual to alter their subtance use behaviour and hence, the associated problems. Based on a disaggregated view of problems, in which it is implicitly assumed that dependence is epiphenomenal, public education campaigns and legislative controls (such as increasing liquor taxation, and controls on drug availability) aim to reduce problems through a reduction in per capita consumption of substances (Kendell 1979). This represents a more optimistic view of the individual's capacity for change than the harm reduction approaches identified in previous sections. Indeed all change-orientated harm reduction approaches and curative approaches are more optimistic than the palliative approaches. However, this does not represent a simple dichotomy.

Certain change-orientated strategies which fall short of offering cure, can be seen as essentially more optimistic than some of the commonly used curative approaches. For example, there has been a considerable growth in the use of minimal intervention treatments such as self-help manuals (Heather 1989; Heather et al. 1987), and brief cognitive behavioural interventions (Sanchez-Craig *et al.* 1989), and also of interventions in the primary care (Babor *et al.* 1986; Wallace *et al.* 1988; Drummond *et al.* 1990), or general hospital setting (Chick *et al.* 1985). Nevertheless, in spite of a great deal of evidence to suggest that brief therapies are as effective as considerably more intensive in-patient approaches (Miller and Hester 1986*b*), many in the alcoholism treatment field remain pessimistic about the value of the former.

Reality vs denial

Arguably the greatest contribution of epidemiology to the alcohol problems field has been the identification of a considerably greater proportion of the population affected by a severe level of alcohol-related problems, and in need of help, than was previously assumed by the largely addiction focused treatment establishment. Addiction concepts view only a small group of severely affected individuals as being in need of treatment. The epidemiological evidence continues to be denied by the treatment community (Drummond and Edwards 1990). This has meant that in practice there are considerable barriers to seeking help, not least of all, the availability of treatment places. Services are generally geared to assisting only the most severely affected (Drummond 1991). In contrast, recent expansion and 'low threshold' admission policies in treatment services for drug takers in many countries, partly in response to the new and greater problems posed by HIV, have made access to treatment for at least this group, more straightforward.

Such denial by experts in the treatment community can also have a profound effect on public perceptions of the kind of problem which is, or is not, worthy of intervention, which could in turn influence patterns of help seeking. It is not uncommon to encounter even a severely dependent drinker who does not see the need either to seek help, or alter their behaviour, because they do not self-identify with the alcoholic stereotype.

WHICH WAY SHOULD WE GO: TOWARDS PROBLEMS OR TOWARDS ADDICTION?

There are clearly advantages in both problem-focused and addiction- or dependence-focused approaches. A problems framework is inherently more pragmatic as well as being more realistic about the scale of the problem to be tackled. Certain problem-focused strategies could be seen as only partially effective, however, providing palliation for only a narrow range of problems, and having little effect on the severely dependent. Addiction-focused approaches are inherently attractive in that they do not involve the pragmatic compromises of problem-focused treatments. However, evidence that more intensive addiction-focused treatments are more effective than less intensive approaches is lacking. Thus, continued emphasis on the deployment of resources in intensive treatments of this sort, catering for only a small sector of the affected population, denies help to many in need of intervention.

The question, however, should not be seen as involving a choice between these two frameworks and the treatment approaches which they imply. While problems and dependence are clearly different phenomena, they are also related as described in Chapter 4, p. 61 (Drummond). They may occur independently and in different degrees. They, most likely, also interact with one another and with drug consumption. Thus, a treatment approach which may be appropriate for one individual may be quite inappropriate for another.

There is some evidence to support the common-sense view that more severely dependent drinkers will benefit more from intensive treatments than the less dependent (Orford *et al.* 1976). Similar, differential effects have been observed in the treatment of cigarette smokers: heavier smokers (the more nicotine dependent) benefit more from nicotine chewing gum as an aid to stopping than lighter smokers (Russell *et al.* 1980). Prescribing injectable heroin with needles and syringes to an opiate taker who expresses some interest in trying to abstain could be seen as negligent, and yet there is a small but vociferous minority who advocate free availability of currently proscribed drugs on the grounds of pragmatic (but far-fetched and conjectural) harm reduction arguments. Similarly, the denial of treatment to a drug taker who is not prepared to consider complete abstinence and a commitment to lengthy, intensive treatment represents churlish rejection of a legitimate attempt to seek help. However obvious these examples may seem they require experimental confirmation (Miller and Hester, 1986*c*). Experiments aimed at finding such matching effects are still at an early stage.

There is a clear case to be made for greater flexibility and responsiveness to individual needs from treatment agencies (ACMD 1988). This brief review should advise against placing too great a faith in unitary solutions to what represents a complex and multifaceted problem. Flexibility can be viewed on two levels. Flexibility at the agency level requires a willingness to consider engaging in therapeutic activities, which are able to adapt to both individual needs and the broader needs of the community at large. The rigid application of one approach to a narrow population is indefensible. Flexibility is also required at the level of the whole system involved in attempting to alleviate the problems associated with substance use. The recent examples of responsiveness to the changing needs of the drug-taking population with the arrival of HIV (Stimson 1990), represents a striking and valuable example for the whole treatment community. Such flexibility must include a willingness to tolerate, and work in conjunction with, a range of different approaches in the common aim of reducing the harm associated with substance use.

REFERENCES

Advisory Council on the Misuse of Drugs (1988). *AIDS and drug misuse Part 1.* HMSO, London.

Anonymous (1987). No 'alcoholism' please, we're British. *British Journal of Addiction*, **82**, 1059–60.

Anonymous (1990). Drinkers are free to stop. *The Independent*, 25th October, p. 26.

Babor, T. F., Ritson, E. B., and Hodgson, R. J. (1986). Alcohol-related problems in the primary health care setting: a review of early intervention strategies. *British Journal of Addiction*, **81**, 23–46.

Brewer, C., Hussein, R., and Bailey, C. (1988). Opioid withdrawal and naltrexone induction in 48–72 hours with minimal drop-out, using a modification of the naltrexone–clonidine technique. *British Journal of Psychiatry*, **153**, 340–3.

Chick, J., Lloyd, G., and Crombie, E. (1985). Counselling problem drinkers in medical wards: a controlled study. *British Medical Journal*, **290**, 965–7.

Drummond, D. C. (1991). Comprehensive strategies for the therapy of alcoholism: where have we gone wrong? In Kalant, H., Khanna, J. M., and Israel, Y. (eds) *Advances in Biomedical Alcohol Research. Proceedings of the Fifth ISBRA/RSA Congress* Suppl. No. 1. *Alcohol and Alcoholism.*

Drummond, D. C. and Edwards, G. (1990). Dogma, denial and drinking problems. *Lancet*, **336**, 1583–4.

Drummond, D. C., Thom, B., Brown, C., Edwards, G., and Mullan, M. J. (1990). Specialist versus general practitioner treatment of problem drinkers. *Lancet*, **336**, 915–18.

Emrick, C. D. (1975). A review of psychologically oriented treatment of alcoholism: 2. the relative effectiveness of different treatment approaches and the effectiveness of treatment versus no treatment. *Journal of Studies on Alcohol*, **36**, 88–108.

Fingarette, H. (1988). *Heavy drinking: the myth of alcoholism as a disease.* University of California Press, Berkeley.

Gorman, D. M. (1989). Is the 'new' problem drinking concept of Heather & Robertson more useful in advancing our scientific knowledge than the 'old' disease concept? *British Journal of Addiction*, **84**, 843–5.

Heather, N. (1989). Psychology and brief interventions. *British Journal of Addiction*, **84**, 357–70.

Heather, N., Robertson, I., MacPherson, B., Allsop, S., and Fulton, A. (1987). Effectiveness of a controlled drinking self-help manual: 1 year follow-up results. *British Journal of Clinical Psychology*, **26**, 279–87.

Jellinek, E. M. (1952). Phases of alcohol addiction. *Quarterly Journal of Studies on Alcohol*, **13**, 673–84.

Jellinek, E. M. (1960). *The disease concept of alcoholism*. Hillhouse, New Brunswick.
Kendell, R. E. (1979). Alcoholism: a medical or a political problem? *British Medical Journal*, **1**, 367–71.
Kleber, H. (1985). Naltrexone. *Journal of Substance Abuse Treatment*, **2**, 117–222.
Maltzman, I. (1989). A reply to Cook, 'craftsman versus professional: analysis of the controlled drinking controversy'. *Journal of Studies on Alcohol*, **50**, 466–72.
Miller, W. R. and Hester, R. K. (1986*a*). Inpatient alcoholism treatment: who benefits? *American Psychologist*, **41**, 794–805.
Miller, W. R. and Hester, R. K. (1986*b*). Effectiveness of alcoholism treatment: what research reveals. In Miller, W. R. and Heather, N. (eds) *Treating addictive behaviors: processes of change*, pp. 121–74. Plenum, New York.
Miller, W. R. and Hester, R. K. (1986*c*). Matching problem drinkers with optimal treatments. In Miller, W. R., and Heather, N. (eds) *Treating addictive behaviors: processes of change*, pp. 175–204. Plenum, New York.
Orford, J., Oppenheimer, E., and Edwards, G. (1976). Abstinence or control: the outcome for excessive drinkers two years after consultation. *Behaviour Research and Therapy*, **14**, 409–18.
Pattersan, M. (1986). *Hooked? N.E.T.: a New Approach to Drug Cure*. Faber and Faber, London.
Russell, M. A. H., Raw, M., and Jarvis, M. J. (1980). Clinical use of nicotine chewing-gum. *British Medical Journal*, **280**, 1599–602.
Sanchez-Craig, M., Leigh, G., Spivak, K., and Lei, H. (1989). Superior outcome of females over males after brief treatment for the reduction of heavy drinking. *British Journal of Addiction*, **84**, 395–404.
Stimson, G. V. (1990). AIDS and HIV: the challenge for *British drug services*. *British Journal of Addiction*, **85**, 329–39.
Trotter, T. (1804). *An essay, medical, philosophical, and chemical, on drunkenness, and its effects on the human body*. Longman Rees, London.
Wallace, P., Cutler, S., and Haines, A. (1988). Randomised controlled trial of general practitioner intervention in patients with excessive alcohol consumption. *British Medical Journal*, **297**, 663–8.

13

The demands which the problem perspective sets for research

MALCOLM LADER, GRIFFITH EDWARDS, AND D. COLIN DRUMMOND

The idea which for too long held sway, that the exclusive focus for concern relating to misuse of alcohol or drugs should be with 'the addict', is clearly now ripe for abandonment. We have instead to take within our field of vision the much more extensive array of people who at some point in their lives, with some frequency or persistence, with any degree of severity, experience this or that adverse consequence of drinking or drug taking. From that shift in vision many practical implications flow. In the immediately preceding chapters, Reginald Smart and Colin Drummond have examined the significance of this perspective for prevention and for treatment.

Hand in hand with a re-thinking of the way in which those practical and policy issues are to be dealt with, must go a reappraisal of research strategies. A new vision of the cause for concern, of what has to be prevented and of who has to be treated, cannot properly be matched by a research strategy which is still over-determined by yesterday's vision of what we should be worrying about. In this chapter we will therefore seek to identify some of the implications for research which are likely to result, when the focus is broadened from the narrow to the wide angle. We will not attempt to construct an exhaustive list of every possible research topic (shopping lists of that kind are seldom profitable), but will instead try to identify some of the general issues which will need to be addressed as research goes forward toward the ever nearing horizon of the year 2000. It should furthermore be emphasized that what will be sketched out is an examination of some of the possible directions for a further research evolution, rather than any total or abrupt change of investigative directions. The question is how best to build on a considerable existing body of problem-orientated research.

This chapter will largely be structured around discussion of potential research developments within three established traditions — research on social processes of problem definition, and the population level, and the more individual level approaches for studying the genesis of problems. We will not replicate the discussion of problem orientated prevention and treatment research given in Chapters 11 (p. 167) and 12 (p. 179). Shorter attention will then be given to the literature database needs which arise with such an amorphous idea as that set by substance problems, and finally a brief note will be entered on the difficult issues of priority setting and research organization.

RESEARCH ON THE SOCIAL PROCESSES OF PROBLEM DEFINITION

Under this heading we have in mind research directed at the question of why and how societies come to view certain alcohol or drug related issues as problematic. The importance of this theme has emerged repeatedly in earlier chapters of this book, particularly in Levine's analysis of temperance cultures (Chapter 2, p. 15), and Pearson's discussion of illicit drugs (Chapter 7, p. 109). Lader's account of the emergence of 'the tranquillizer problem' (Chapter 10, p. 161), shows how broadly this question runs. If one were looking for even further material it would be possible to find variations on this same theme in relation to tobacco, as for instance in the recent growth of concern over passive smoking (Raw *et al.* 1990). Comparisons between different substances, across cultures and across time, will provide a strong research strategy, with studies perhaps being conducted not only on how behaviour comes to be seen as problematic, but also the converse. How does a society succeed in turning a persistently blind eye toward what the public health activist may view as a manifest and neglected problem?

It is easy to dismiss the study of why a country or an era deems a particular behaviour to be something to worry about, as potentially only rather 'soft science', as an optional extra, an issue likely to attract no more than yet another reflex application of labelling theory, or provide a playground for conspiracy theorists. The authors would argue very much otherwise, and would assert that there are questions here of great social importance which deserve further and sustained attention from historians and social scientists (MacAndrew and Edgerton 1969). There are many examples already of scholarly analysis in this kind of area (the considerable literature which has grown up around Prohibition for instance e.g. Gusfield 1986, Blocker 1989, or the historical studies which have been published on national and international movements towards opium and 'narcotic' control e.g. Musto 1973; Berridge and Edwards 1981). One is still though left with the conclusion that there is a great range of further issues of this type, both historical and more recent, which will repay scrutiny. Indeed, for the ambitious young scholar who is seeking a thesis topic there is the allure here of a relatively uncrowded territory, and the chance of finding primary sources which have not as yet been repeatedly thumbed over by other aspiring Ph.D. students.

PROBLEMS RESEARCH AT POPULATION LEVEL

The genesis of problems: consumption and dependence

Much recent epidemiological research in the alcohol field has been directed at the relationship between population consumption levels and rates of problem experience, and findings of crucial importance to prevention and public health have emerged (Bruun *et al.* 1975). The demonstration of a dose–response relationship between number of cigarettes smoked and morbidity and mortality, also exemplifies the importance of research which essentially focuses on a two-variable analysis (Doll and Hill 1950). With illicit drugs it is though difficult to think of any very extensive application of that model.

Let us for illustrative purposes focus for a moment on findings from the alcohol sector. What has essentially been show here is that at the population level, more drink generally means more problems, and less drink less problems. Give or take a little, and for a variety of indicators, this conclusion is robust across populations and across time (Schmidt 1977). The results which Colin Drummond presents in Chapter 4 do however begin to suggest that further insights will in certain circumstances be gained if dependence is put into the analysis as a third variable. If that suggestion is correct, questions then open up for problems research of a quite complex nature. Given that in a clinical population, dependence has important mediating implications for understanding the relationship between consumption and problems (Drummond 1990), to what degree is this same consideration likely to bear on non-clinical populations, and the interpretation of findings from community samples? Furthermore, if dependence complicates or distorts the consumption/problems connections, what may in turn be the relationship between different consumption patterns and the likely proportion of the population contracting dependence of any degree? Animal work suggests that continued rather intermittent exposure is a more effective schedule for instating dependence (Edwards 1990).

Different substances have of course different dependence potentials, and also diverse capacities to produce harm. The consumption/dependence/problems connection may therefore involve different equations with different weightings for different classes of drugs, and cross-substance comparisons may again provide an interesting research strategy. But whatever the substance, one emerging argument may be that research on the consumption/problems connection will be handicapped if it leaves habit or dependence out of the reckoning.

The personal and contextual variables

Consumption may be the old star and dependence a possibly important new actor in the problems play, but one of the strong messages that comes through several of the foregoing chapters is that in explaining the genesis of problems at population level, it remains very necessary also to seek further understanding of the contributions made by a wide range of other variables which are far from mere bit actors. Some of these variables can be subsumed under a 'personal' heading, while others can be described as 'contextual', but as Lee Robins argues in Chapter 8 (p. 133), the distinction between the two categories is not absolute. Research on all these issues seems amply and repeatedly to demonstrate their importance, and one may indeed experience a certain sense of ennui when yet another study demonstrates that, say, childhood behaviour disorder or socio-economic deprivation are predictors of drug problems. The challenge to problem orientated research must continue to be that of getting beyond the associations to explaining the process.

Survey databases as a valuable commodity

Talk at the abstract level about the importance of this kind of survey research is all very well, but who is going to undertake the actual work? We not only need large-scale and representative cross-sectional samples, but must hope that there will be resources to repeat some of these surveys at regular five year intervals. At best there will also be support for research which will allow repeat interviewing of the same cohorts over time: for certain questions, longitudinal research is indispensable.

Thus the hard fact of the matter is that many of the intriguing questions that are raised in this book are at present only likely to be systematically tackled in a very few countries which possess the necessary resources, expertise, and commitment, and even that may be an optimistic assessment. In Britain there is certainly a need to obtain better national data on alcohol and drug use and related problems.

Data sets which can be used to test the questions raised above constitute, therefore, a valuable and all too scant commodity. The research community would benefit from a system which gave an updated index of archival data sets on an international basis.

Statistical and logical issues

A strong inference to be drawn from Skog's dissection of questions around the nature of causality (Chapter 3, p. 37), is that we should be cautious about the assumptions which lurk in the phrases 'alcohol related' or 'drug related'. Further investment in the analysis of the logical assumptions involved in population level problems research is needed. We are perhaps too readily and too often imputing cause from association in highly complex multi-variate fields, with a tendency also to draw generalized conclusions from very special data sets. The pressure to produce 'findings', seems inimicable to anyone devoting adequate time and funding to the hard logical critique which is needed if we are better to know which findings are golden, and which are mere fool's gold.

Theory

With a rich research experience on which to build, with much empirical data gathered, and with better data sets and more hope of cross-national and cross-substance comparisons, with further longitudinal studies, with perhaps a strengthening of the logic and statistics, with all this and much more, one clear further message from what the contributors to this book are telling, is that we will get nowhere without a strengthening of theory. The earliest surveying tradition in this field was frankly and joyously empirical (e.g. Cahalan 1970). Since then little bits of theory have been proposed, and on occasion more fully articulated theories (Skog 1986). It would be immensely worthwhile if over the next decade, some stronger, more integrative, testable, and competing theories were to emerge. This may well be a prime area for collaborative thinking between different disciplines — economists, sociologists, psychologists, and (if dependence enters the population level equations), the pharmacologists and biological scientists. Who knows, Tim Peters' dream (Chapter 9, p. 151) of 'one science' may in the process become real.

PROBLEMS RESEARCH AT THE INDIVIDUAL LEVEL

The segmentation between population and individual level approaches to investigating the genesis of substance problems is arbitrary, but under this heading we will consider the kind of research which is concerned with relatively small patient or subject groups, and animal research. Such investigations seek to go beyond the probabilistic statements of the large population studies, and explore the characteristics or circumstances of the individual as bearing on the likelihood of a problem being individually contracted.

Tim Peters' chapter (Chapter 9, p. 151) exemplifies this kind of approach so far as the biological study of alcohol-induced myositis is concerned. The biological component to alcohol problems research has over recent years made important connections with genetic research. One can probably assume that work of this kind now has its considerable momentum and will find its own way forward, but there are still enormously important problems to be addressed in relation to a range of common and destructive alcohol related tissue pathologies, including brain damage, liver disease, pancreatitis, and fetal damage (Secretary of Health and Human Services 1990). So far as illicit drugs are concerned, HIV infection has become the issue of overwhelming importance, but the consequent research questions must relate not only to the characteristics of the virus but also to the multiple determinants of the individual behaviour which leads to use of the dirty equipment, unsafe sex, and the risk of virus infection. Although HIV is today the problem at centre stage, there are still many other questions relating to drug induced physical complications or tissue pathologies which deserve research attention, whether in relation to opiates, cocaine, 'designer drugs', or benzodiazepines.

The study of problems in the psychological and social domain at the individual level lies a long way from the technologies and neat experimental designs of the more biological type of problems research, and here there are still some classic questions waiting for an answer. Why does one sibling in a family or even the identical twin develop a drinking problem, but not the other? What are the protective factors which enable a teenager to avoid involvement in drug use when many of his or her peers are using heroin? What is the real nature of the alcohol–crime nexus, or the relationship between alcohol and family violence? There is thus a long list of good 'problem' questions at individual level which continue to stand in need of good research design. The value of observational and qualitative research should not be forgotten, and it is a mistake to put too much faith in the supposedly conclusive quantitative research approach in the hope that it will provide the all time and generalizable answer. We may, as it were, in problems research do better sometimes to rest with individual level research which yields truth for the particular village.

PROBLEMS RESEARCH AND ITS LITERATURE NEEDS

The past twenty years has seen an exponential increase in the amount of published scientific material, and research on substance problems has participated in this trend. The field covers such a range of disciplines that a large number of publications need to be scanned. Access to an up-to-date and well organized literature database is essential.

Reference databases are only as good as their keywords, the tags which are attached to each paper entered into the system. The choice of such keywords is thus an important matter and bibliographers need the assistance of professionals in the field. That this is not yet standard is evidenced by the typical literature research, where one is either inundated by marginally relevant references or ends up with almost none.

Formulating research in terms of problems compounds this difficulty. Key words usually comprise concrete terms, and problems may not be easily distilled into such terms. Wider concepts like dependence are too broad to be helpful. In the end each researcher may need to develop his own system, using a common database but attaching his own keywords. Modern personal computers are quite capable of coping with such a system.

Such databases deal only with published material. It is also essential to know what research is in the pipeline nationally and internationally. Congresses and conferences are the traditional ways of doing this. In addition, there are compendia of ongoing research which are published regularly in certain countries.

PRIORITY SETTING AND THE ORGANIZATION OF PROBLEM RESEARCH

As mentioned earlier, it has not been the authors' purpose to set out a shopping list of problems which they believe to be of the highest priority. Rather, it is their wish to emphasize that several factors should enter into the equation, establishing the degree of priority of the study. It is important that as many viewpoints as possible contribute to the debate on the importance of a problem. Who could have forecast that unexplained infections in Central Africa in the early 1980s would have become a pandemic of AIDS a few years later, and have transformed our attitudes to injecting users of illicit drugs? If more notice had been taken of the mode of transmission of the HIV virus, steps to limit its spread among addict populations might have been taken earlier.

Feasibility must always be an issue when setting priorities. The degree of sophistication involved in the relevant techniques is another important factor. Many questions cannot be answered because techniques are not available in man, or are relatively crude. The study of the relationship between mood changes and alcohol use remains largely on a descriptive rather than an analytical level because we have no sensitive techniques to measure the biochemical changes accompanying anxiety and depression.

The study of effective remedies can sometimes provide a useful handle on understanding dating mechanisms. If a therapeutic manipulation is shown to be effective using rigorous criteria, then exploring the mechanism of action of the manipulation *may* throw light on the underlying condition. But it may not, as the therapy may act on a totally separate mechanism, either in parallel with or sequentially beyond the abnormality associated with the alcohol drug pathology.

The organization of problem oriented research

Much research can profitably be pursued by individuals or small groups of individuals. Each can identify a problem, to find it and refine it to the point where a testable hypothesis can be made. But then help may be needed to devise the survey or experiment, apply the technique, and analyse the data. As research on alcohol, drug, and nicotine problems either at population or individual level becomes more complex, the possibility that any small group, let alone an individual, will have all those skills available becomes more and more remote. It is thus essential that advice and expertise are available both within and without this special field. Larger units are essential in order to provide the critical mass to pursue this kind of research success fully. There is an increasingly important place for collaboration, networking, and bringing in high level expertise from parent disciplines.

The technique-orientated side of things is more problematic. The substance research experts themselves must seek advice and help from the people from the centres of excellence who are using the new techniques. By a process of successive iteration, the problem and the technique can be locked together. However, the substance experts will then find themselves having to trust their technical colleagues entirely with respect to the data quality, and the technical experts will have to trust their colleagues in the applied field not to get them to expend resources on a trivial problem.

Multi-disciplinary teams are generally regarded as the best way to promote research in complex areas such as we are talking about here and in other parts of this book. Nevertheless, the most invaluable person is the one who is able to cross the disciplinary boundaries and talk sensibly to his colleagues in two or more disciplines. If he can identify problems as well and apply appropriate techniques, then the topic will prosper.

REFERENCES

Berridge, V. and Edwards, G. (1981). *Opium and the people; opiate use in nineteenth century England.* Allen Lane, London.

Blocker, J. S. (1989). *American temperance movements: cycles of reform.* Twayne, Boston.

Bruun, K., Edwards, G., Lumio, M., Mäkelä, K., Pan, L., Popham, R. E., et al. (1975). *Alcohol control policies in public health perspective.* Finnish Foundation for Alcohol Studies, Helsinki.

Cahalan, D. (1970). *Problem drinkers.* Jossey Bass, San Francisco.

Doll, R. and Hill, A. B. (1950). Smoking and carcinoma of the lung. *British Medical Journal,* ii, 739–48.

Drummond, D. C. (1990). The relationship between alcohol dependence and

alcohol-related problems in a clinical population. *British Journal of Addiction*, **85**, 357–66.
Edwards, G. (1990). Withdrawal symptoms and alcohol dependence; fruitful mysteries. *British Journal of Addiction*, **85**, 447–61.
Gusfield, J. R. (1986). *Symbolic crusade: status politics and the American Temperance Movement* (2nd edn). University of Illinois Press, Urbana.
MacAndrew, C. and Edgerton, R. (1969). *Drunken comportment: a Societal Explanation.* Aldine, Chicago.
Musto, D. F. (1973). *The American disease: origins of narcotic control.* Yale University Press, New Haven.
Raw, M., White, P., and McNeill, A. (1990). *Clearing the air; a guide for action tobacco.* British Medical Association, London.
Schmidt, W. (1977). Cirrhosis and alcohol consumption: an epidemiological perspective. In Edwards, G. and Grant, M. (eds) *Alcoholism; new knowledge and new responses,* Chap. 1, pp. 15–47. Croom Helm, London.
Secretary of Health and Human Services (1990). *Alcohol and health; Seventh Special Report to the US Congress.* US Department of Health and Human Services, Rockville, Massachusetts.
Skog, O.-J. (1986). The long waves of alcohol consumption: A social network perspective on cultural change. *Social Networks*, **8**, 1–32.
Strang, J. and Stimson, S. (1990). *AIDS and drug misuse.* Routledge, London.

14

The meanings of problem: a debate around a problematic concept

The second day of the Cumberland Lodge meeting from which this book derives, was devoted entirely to debate. Give or take a little movement in and out of the room, the participants numbered about twenty and they are listed on pp. ix and x. Among these discussants were clinicians working in both statutory and voluntary agencies, administrators, and research scientists drawn from such varied backgrounds as sociology, the history and philosophy of science, biological medicine, psychopharmacology, and psychosocial aspects of psychiatry.

The discussion focused on the nature of 'problem' as a concept, and more specifically on the concept of 'substance-related problem'. The intimacy of a small group (and the setting of a book-lined room with views over Windsor Great Park), the mix of practitioners and scientists, the perspectives brought by different countries, and the cross-cutting of ideas drawn from experiences with licit and illicit substance use, led to a rich mix of arguments. By close of play, probably everyone who had been involved in the debate felt that difficult questions had been usefully and unusually forced out of the shadows. 'Problem' is a word often too easily nodded through as if we all really know what the word means — an 'it's obvious' kind of response. What this debate demonstrated is that 'substance problem' is a concept meaning many different things to different people. To assume its 'obviousness' may result in 'obvious' policy solutions that are ill-judged. Hence, time spent on sorting out ideas is likely to be time well-spent.

The transcript of this discussion ran to a total of 130 typed pages, and the editorial problem has been to find how best to distil the essence but at the same time retain the sharp sense of debate. We wanted to let the reader feel that he or she too was personally involved in the discussion, but without reproducing an extended Hansard type of report of almost monograph length. The discussants seem to have had an astonishing word output per minute, with the social scientists certainly showing in this regard the greatest productivity. The editors finally decided that the best way of proceeding was to identify certain main themes, and then use carefully selected quotations to illustrate them.

'A PROBLEM IS NOT A SCIENTIFIC CONCEPT'

At the start of the debate the view was offered that 'problem' is, in this particular arena, such a shifting, amorphous, and socially loaded concept as to be unlikely usefully to serve scientific discourse in any way.

Dr Skog: A problem is not fundamentally a scientific concept; cirrhosis is a scientific concept and aggression is a scientific concept. With regard to problems, shorthand terms are still used in scientific surveys covering a lot of different consequences, a situation which I do not like. Let us take suicide as an example. Typically one would say that suicide is a negative consequence of something, but there have existed, and probably still do exist, cultures that in specific circumstances would consider suicide a very honourable way of dying. Thus there are at least particular subclasses of suicide that would not be considered to be a problem. Is dependence a problem? I am strongly dependent on coffee. It can keep me going for 12 hours at the computer, and I think that is a good thing. It is the kind of dependence I value although my wife may say it is a problem because I work too much. What is a problem is to a large extent a matter of context and opinion, and of the level we are talking about — the individual, a group, or society at large. If we count 'problem' as a scientific concept there should exist an objective method for deciding whether this specimen of behaviour belongs to that category. I do not think this kind of method exists. One could think about the majority view; is there a consensus in society about what is a problem or whether one particular type of behaviour is a problem? If so, normally it will vary a lot over time. In Norway we are now repeating a survey that was done 25 years ago in which we described different types of drinking behaviour. We asked people, 'Do you consider this to be a problem? Is this abuse or not?' In the 25 years there have been dramatic changes in how people define alcohol abuse and alcohol problems in Norway. Drinking behaviours that years ago were considered a problem by 70 per cent of the population, are now considered so by only 30 per cent. Furthermore, it is very difficult to rely on the concept of a majority decision where multidimensional questions are involved.

Dr Ravetz: Is this change in Norway in the direction of greater or lesser permissiveness toward drunken behaviour?

Dr Skog: More permissive.

Although the group accepted Skog's fundamental point that the concept of problem is 'a matter of context and opinion', the consensus view was that it is still a concept which, for the social scientist, serves very well as a starting point for enquiry. How does 'context and opinion', shape or construct 'problem'? What is the relationship between external reality and social construct?

Dr Ghodse: I fully agree with Dr Skog, and I do not see a 'problem' as a scientific concept. It is not quantifiable. It varies according to the observer. It is culture- and time-bound. It is not an all or nothing phenomenon. It emerges and fades away. Although it is not a scientific concept this does not mean that it is not a useful concept.

Dr Ravetz suggested that 'a problem is a construct reflecting on certain realities.'

THE SOCIAL PROCESSES THAT CONSTRUCT PROBLEMS OUT OF SUBSTANCE USE

The discussion identified a number of social processes which may lead to the use of a psychoactive substance being deemed problematic. For instance, one suggestion was that a problem is an unwanted event plus the sense of a feasible alternative.

Mr Woodcock: There is a tendency to talk indiscriminately about all unwanted effects of drugs as 'problems'. A problem is an unwanted effect plus the demand that something should be done about it. People are of course often unwilling to label an unwanted effect a problem until they can see that there is an alternative. The unwanted effects of barbiturates were not viewed as a problem by the medical profession until the benzodiazepines came along and there was an alternative. Then very quickly the medical profession said, 'Barbiturates are a terrible problem, we must stop prescribing them'.

Another approach was to see 'problem' as a deviation from an ideal.

Dr MacGregor: The common element that we are talking about is something that has to do with adverse effects. When we take the notion of adverse effect in terms of either the individual or society, we are contrasting the notion of a problem with something that is not a problem. In the individual therefore, we are talking about a lack of health or disease, as compared with something called healthy living and a healthy body. The same assumptions arise when discussing a social problem. We are contrasting a problem in society with some notion of social order, or a well balanced society, or a regulated society. We must always look at what the opposite is to the problem, what concept we have in mind in our practice and our theories which we counterpoise to the notion of a problem.

Discussion also centred around the extent to which society defines problems not in terms of the drug or its consequences, but who is using the drug — young people, women, ethnic minorities, and so on.

Dr Bewley: Sometimes people use a word when they mean something else. For example, some years ago in the United States when people talked about the 'heroin addiction problem', that was shorthand; what they meant was the 'young male black crime problem'.

Mr Woodcock: Yes, it is often not a question of what the drug does, but who is using it. One can go back to Troy Duster with his theory that in the United States opiate use did not become perceived as a problem until it was seen to be a matter not of respectable middle-aged women consuming medicines, but of lower class men taking opiates in an addictive way. This fits in with the question of power, and who is saying what the problem is. There is a strong element of those with power and privilege tending to regard an activity which they feel is quite acceptable among their own class, as a problem when it is engaged in by others.

A challenge to the view that the powerful always impose their definition of drug misuse on the powerless by *force majeure*, was though also entered.

Dr Pearson: One entirely legitimate issue particularly where questions of illicit drugs are concerned is the impact that drug use has on the wider community. I raise this only to point to the fact that this is not at all uncommonly an area of silence in the discussions of clinicians and associated researchers. It also means that there is a silence about enforcement. If one's concern is essentially directed towards the good of the patient and his or her family, it worries me that one may be in danger of forgetting the legitimate community concerns. If you are living in a socially deprived neighbourhood that has suffered not only the ravages of econmic deprivation and housing decay, but also a heroin epidemic, you have a right to define heroin as a problem.

Indeed, in the USA there has at times been no group with a stronger anti-heroin position than the Black Panther movement.

As regards making problems out of medically prescribed psychotropics, one element which it was suggested might sometimes be at work was the search for a lost Utopian drug-free innocence.

Dr Kreitman: The issue we have started to look at is: what is wrong with the position of the stable user of a psychotropic drug, which appears to produce no intrinsic effects in itself until it is withdrawn; what is wrong with a state of mild dependency? When that becomes seen as 'a problem', then behind that designation as a problem is a set of moral values. It is of interest just to list the suggestions as to what those values might be. Sometimes the drug may be construed as a substitute for action, and the 'problem' comes about because it is morally preferable if the individual takes arms against a sea of troubles rather than taking yet another tablet.

It may also be sensible to be wary of taking a substance for many years if it could lead to consequences which are as yet unknown, so why take the chance? However, I think there is at least a third theme which comes as a kind of arcadian myth which is increasingly powerful in our society. This relates to the general sense that we have all arrived in a technologically complex and potentially damaging environment, and we ought to get back to the state of the noble savage as quickly as we possibly can. We should take a hostile view of technology; we should eat only potatoes grown in organic compost; we should avoid all E substances. And somehow we are led to adopt almost an anti-scientific stand. I have been concerned at times at the growth among young people of interests in astrology, various kind of naturism, and things that at one time we might all have thought rather cranky. There is a mythological level of wanting once again to be a milkmaid in the dairy, churning butter rather than buying food. Drugs of all kinds are bad because they are 'unnatural'.

'DRUG PROBLEMS' AS A SCREEN TO AVOID LOOKING AT THE PROBLEMS WHICH LIE BEHIND THE DRUG USE

The drug problem might not be just a 'shorthand' for 'young male black crime', but a surface focus which allows society very conveniently to avoid seeing or dealing with certain uncomfortable and deeper problems, which may underlie a community's propensity to use drugs.

Dr Levine: One answer has always been, if only they were to get their hands on less of the stuff — whether the stuff be alcohol or other drugs — then they would have less problems. That has been the major public health approach in the field. There is though another approach which is more sociological. It is that the social conditions often produce the drug problems. In America today it seems to be obvious that 'crack' users tend to be poor, and in New York and other cities they tend to be non-white; they tend to be young; they tend to be people from families and neighbourhoods and schools which have little going for them, and they feel their lives are closed and dead-ended. The obvious solution is to address those underlying problems. That is an explicit policy call. It is both Utopian and, I think, practical at the same time.

Another speaker instanced the epidemiological distribution of suicide as pointing to the same general issue.

Dr Kreitman: This comes on to Harry Levine's point about social deprivation. We have spent a lot of time in my own research group looking at a different issue, the relationship of long-term unemployment to suicide. Sporadically requests come from WHO or other circles saying, 'What kind of a policy can be adopted to reduce suicide?'. One of the things we say is, 'The long term unemployment variable appears to make quite a substantial contribution, and the solution therefore is to avoid long-term unemployment'. That is not a message which governments are prepared to hear. If we look at overdoses and parasuicide, we say, 'There are rates of prevalence of parasuicide seven times higher in areas of the city which can be defined by census indicators of deprivation. We can suggest therapeutic regimes once people have taken overdoses, but if you are interested in prevention then the kind of strategy you should adopt is to reduce deprivation'. They do not want to hear this, but they do want the research to be done in order to keep the academics happy, and to be able to show and claim that a liberal approach has been taken and all avenues are being examined. But I would maintain that it is partly in order not to hear the result. I do not think that is naive.

Levine referred to the general category of 'politically inconvenient knowledge', but another speaker evinced some pity for the politicians.

Dr Kidger: You can move in two directions. The first direction is towards a solution to the problem at personal level. As clinicians, that is our orientation. We are carers; we like to see a personal solution. You also can move backwards towards causality, which equals responsibility, which equals blame. I have no difficulty in understanding why people should find it difficult to accept the explanation of a problem if the blame ends up on their lap. I do not see it as difficult to understand why a government might find it difficult to accept that unemployment is causing addiction problems. That may explain why at the moment the biological and genetic explanations for addiction are so attractive; they do not leave the blame sitting on anyone's lap. Who ends up with the blame is one of the most important social consequences of any problem model.

THE SCIENTIST'S VIEW AND THE DRUG USER'S VIEW OF THE NATURE OF THE PROBLEM MAY NOT ALWAYS BE IN SYNCHRONY

All too easily, it was suggested, scientists may impose on the field their own views as to what counts as the problem.

Dr Pearson: It is easy to lose awareness that scientists and practitioners are, all the time, actively involved in defining 'the problem'. It is as if all that we are doing is routinely to carry out research, routinely treat patients, within whatever set of moral, political or policy prescriptions are defined elsewhere. I simply want to say that this is not true. On the one hand, all these people are shaping policy, both through formal arrangements in a whole variety of advisory committees, and in terms of their interventions in professional societies. They even help to frame Parliamentary legislation. There are these many formal channels of influence. In addition, both historians and social scientists would say that even in the routine, informal activities of scientists and practitioners, by the nature of the questions that they ask, and by the very nature of the questions that they choose to ignore, they are engaged in the practice of defining problems.

Ms Milburn: We must consider how individuals who are using various substances themselves define or do not define their use as a problem. What one sees with illegal drugs is that usually their use is defined as a problem most powerfully by external people, by relations, by friends, by the legal system, and that tends often to come before any clear internal definition of the problem. What usually characterizes the individual relationship with the substance is a feeling of ambivalence.

Dr Hore: The patients' problem is often simply how he or she *feels*, a matter of undifferentiated anxiety.

Geoffrey Pearson then came in again with a strong plea for listening to what the drug users themselves not only see as a problem, but what they may insist is not problematic at all.

Dr Pearson: Supposing some young social scientist comes back and tells you this. He says, 'You define drug misuse at the moment as a war on drugs, or a problem of law and order, as this or that, but I want to tell you that I have been standing out there in the rain, I have been hanging around outside youth clubs, sitting patiently in pharmacists shops, keeping notes about the exchanges of young bedraggled men and women who come in and out, having conversations with them, and what I want to say to you is that you have completely got the problem wrong. I want to reformulate this problem as one in which young people are engaged in an activity in which the fraternal nature of that lifestyle involves a great many high risk activities, in particular sharing injecting equipment, placing them at high risk of both contracting and assisting in the transmission of the AIDS epidemic. Therefore, as a scientist, I wish my science to define policy, and the orientation of practice, and the investment of resources, and the definition of the problem, in entirely different ways from the perspective in which they are at the moment conceived.'

Dr Ghodse: What is it that is so special about drugs just because they are mind-acting? We know there are considerable problems in the use of antibiotics, and there has been irrational use of antibiotics with harmful consequences. Similar examples are numerous and we know, for example, that there has been highly irrational use of vitamins. What is so peculiar about psychoactive drugs that we make out of them such a big 'problems' agenda?

STUDYING PROBLEMS: WHAT SORT OF SCIENCE IS NEEDED?

One lone, bold and heterodox challenge, was put to the expected consensus view that the study of drug problems has to be a multidisciplinary undertaking with a strengthened social science emphasis.

Dr Peters: Biochemically, I think there is one science: I do not think there are separate sciences. We have seen this in psychology, how it has moved toward physiological and molecular psychology. The same thing will happen in sociology. In the next decade we can expect the emergence of a molecular and biochemical sociology.

Some other views on the balance of needed sciences were these.

Mr Turner: What we tend to do is to concentrate on the dependence or the problem at a very individual, personal level. Somehow we have to break that mould. We have generally been poor at picking up on the sociological side of these questions. Perhaps this is because, for historical reasons, we have defined the problem down into a single medical discipline with various branches, and almost separated ourselves from the context of the problem with which we are dealing. Until we escape from that position, we shall not influence policy because we have in fact defined ourselves out of involvement in the policy process.

Dr Raistrick: We must consider research at two levels, a social level and an individual level. We can make some kinds of statement about the consequences of having available certain drugs, with certain populations, in certain conditions. Within some sort of dialogue between researchers and policy-makers, we can come to a reasonable idea about what type of controls it might be reasonable to impose on society as a whole, so that harm is kept to an acceptable level and a reasonable balance struck between damage to society and individual freedom. If we look at things more at an individual level, it is more difficult. I am not sure how all the different sciences come to bear to explain problem formation at the individual level. The clinician is the person who, more as artist than as scientist, is good at plucking a bit from this and a bit from that and saying, 'That seems to fit; maybe that would be a useful thing to bring to bear to prevent or treat this particular individual problem'.

Dr Drummond: There is an important point in trying to understand who determines science policy. Across the Atlantic it seems that science policy in addictions is moving more towards a biological model than it has been in previous years, and projects that look at genetics and at the fundamental physiological processes, seem increasingly to be preferred to studies that look more at the social and psychological causes of alcohol and drug problems. This has the effect of blocking research that could broaden the debate. When research is focused on predominantly biological issues, the general public starts to develop the impression that this is what is really important about drug problems, and begins to ignore social issues. Research of this kind is actually influencing people's perception of the problem.

These concerns about what kinds of science, in what degree of mix, are most likely to elucidate the nature of substance problems (and produce science which can speak effectively to policy), were then put in a wider context by an intervention which probably persuaded everyone present that there are advantages in bringing to any specialized debate on drugs the fresh breeze of ideas from the outside.

Dr Ravetz: In this area we are engaged in what Kuhn would probably call prescience. Kuhn distinguishes between pure sciences, which are based on a model of mathematical experimental sciences, and all the others which are less mature. Having myself been a professional historian I do not like that pecking order. History got going as a discipline in late eighteenth century Germany when the experimental sciences were still rather amateur affairs. The English language concept of 'science' is very restrictive. If you go to the Slavic cultures you have a term which includes poetry, and maybe even the visual arts. In every area of activity there are people doing something which can be described as some kind of problem solving activity. There are techniques for writing poetry and writing music; one can distinguish between good and bad poetry and good and bad musical compositions. What comes out is not at all like physics, but then even physics is culturally conditioned. In the Renaissance, it was certainly considered that a painting conveyed truth in the same way as the invention of a machine or the discovery of a scientific law. I tend to be much more ecumenical in my ideas on what constitutes science, perhaps to validate my own professional position. The question then would be: given any problem area, such as addiction, what is the best way to solve problems. The issue, I think, is not so much, are we scientists when we look at addiction, but are we doing the best that we can? There is clearly a broad agreement that we need clinicians and biochemists, and we need historians. Again I am reminded of where Aristotle pointed out that every field of enquiry has its appropriate methods and its appropriate degree of precision in results. He says, 'You would not want to use rhetoric in a geometrical argument, but neither would you want to use geometry for an ethical argument'. This is a very important point but we tend to forget it. For various cultural reasons we have a situation where, physics being taken as the model, other sciences validate themselves by trying to be like physics. Among some philosophers of science they use the term 'physics envy', with its obvious psychoanalytical connotations. It is therefore possible to hyperquantify, make the activity much like physics, when that is inappropriate for the study in hand. I see the task of a philosopher as being more to characterize and help people in the management of the inherent uncertainties of their fields, rather than to find rules whereby certainty can be achieved. When we realize that there are insoluble contradictions we can interpret what we are doing at the scientific level in a more enriched and realistic way. To hope we can have one simple physics of addiction which will then pour out results for the policy makers, is vain.

The proper concerns of science in this field should not, one speaker further suggested, be prematurely constrained by a two dimensional framework.

Dr Madden: We should move beyond two axes, as has been done with psychiatric classification. Level of consumption is an axis that we should note. We might also split the problem axis into the organic problems, and social and psychological problems. Tobacco is high on a scale for producing organic problems and rather low on social problems. Many of the opiates, at least when taken by non-injection methods, would score in the reverse order. Another scale would be the cultural factors. That could be split into the macro features of society, and the immediate environment. You might consider that the economic factors are sufficiently understood to warrant an axis independent, or that the moral and religious factors warrant an axis of their own split away from the broader cultural factors. The dependence potential of a drug is another axis. A final dimension is the genetic predisposition. Again there are two aspects within that, genetic vulnerability to dependence and vulnerability to the organic complications of dependence. I would therefore make a plea for a science of more dimensions than we have developed so far.

In this debate around research, a final note, query, or provocation, was entered thus.

Dr Lader: In this day and age when we have to allocate priorities, one factor which weighs is whether anything is an 'interesting problem'. What do we mean by 'interesting problem'? Do we mean it is of interest to a lot of people and therefore a common problem; do we mean it is of interest to the scientist; do we mean it is interesting because it is susceptible to an elegant solution? I think it is almost the latter. Something can be regarded by scientists as interesting not because the problem is interesting, but because the solution is regarded as elegant.

SUBSTANCE PROBLEMS, AND HOW IS SCIENCE TO SPEAK TO POLICY?

How is science in this particular arena to influence policy? That question is no doubt only in some respects special to substance problems, with the basic science/policy question far more general. One issue already touched on above was the possibility that in this area (as elsewhere), the scientific findings may not necessarily be welcome on the policy maker's lap. In a section of the debate which seemed at times to be coloured by despair, the following more cheerful note was entered.

Dr Bewley: I was feeling gloomy about this session and thought we might be studying the wrong things; that, since we have no effect on policymakers, we ought probably to be studying the inward workings of chancellors. But I remembered that science in this field has at times brought about changes in policies. One example would be the publication of the Wootton Report on cannabis which was very unwelcome at the time, both to government and the opposition, because it was not what they wanted to hear. Since then, what was recommended in that report has in effect been generally accepted. This is an example where the giving of good scientifically based advice on a 'drug problem', (even though it was not accepted at the time), did affect the development of policy later on.

A view which was not so much contradictory as tangential was however also put: it may be possible radically to effect a policy change with surprisingly little underpinning from science.

Ms Milburn: I have been turning over in my mind what has gone on in the last three or four years in terms of treatment and policy responses to injecting drug users, and how HIV and AIDS have changed this scene. There has been a sea change in the way that services are organized. I am not at all certain what the influence of research has been on that change: there was a change in practice and policy that came into play much more quickly than I have seen in other areas in the last 15 or so years. What has science had to do with all this?

Instance after instance was however identified where research had pointed toward an effective preventive remedy, but policy makers had not wanted to hear the message.

Dr Pearson: A rather more belligerent profession might for instance say, 'We are tired of engaging in this pretty blue-skies research on alcohol. We will refuse to do any research whatsoever until you take notice of what we have already said to you on a common-sense level, which is, 'Do something about national levels of alcohol consumption, whether through taxation policy, or whatever'. It is a paradox that we are funded for doing all kinds of rather intricate basic work and yet we already have a body of knowledge which would point quite clearly in a very practical policy direction.

Dr Ravetz: Policy is not science.

Dr MacGregor: We should think about the question of to whom we talk. We have perhaps been made rather complacent and lazy by expecting that we would have the ear of government, and government would listen to what we said. Government is not the only audience. We should not just talk to government, but should accept a responsibility to engage in public debate. I believe in this strategy for two reasons. Firstly, quite often we have more information and a better judgement than many of those whose voices are strong in decision-making. Secondly, there is an issue where I think medicine and the professions in general have something to offer, and that is to do with ethics. This is where the practitioners in particular come in. We are not just talking about science, although there is an ethics of science. We are talking about professional ethics. There is something involved in professional ethics, a set of values which should bear on decision making. We believe in the relief of suffering — and that is valuable. I would encourage us not to despair.

CONCLUSION: A DEBATE THAT NEEDS TO BE WIDELY CONTINUED

This chapter has tried to show how a particular group of people attempted on a particular day to grapple with the 'meanings of problem' question. Far from there being any immodest presumption that this group could produce an uniquely incisive analysis of epic finality, we would suggest that very evidently they do no more than identify a few starting points. The only firm conclusion at this juncture is that the kind of debate started here does indeed deserve to be taken further in wider forums, with a different mix of intellects, with other types of erudition, and many another fresh breeze. Science may be poetry, sociology may be biochemistry in an immature form (or vice versa), the bedraggled young people have much to tell, we must go on funding the politically inconvenient, the 'problem' concept is difficult to make into science but on present showing it is a good start for argument.

Index

abstinence 6, 184
abuse 37–59, 91, 94–5, 133–50, 161
  alcohol 15, 17, 87–94, 151–60, 200
  drug 87, 89, 93, 145, 163–4, 173
accidents 64, 89, 92, 102, 168–70
acetaldehyde 151–4, 157
addiction 7, 8, 26, 68, 204
  bi-axial concept 62, 63, 70, 72, 79
  definition of 1, 4, 61, 85–7, 92, 161, 179
  treatment of 180–1, 185–7
  see also dependence; problem/s
adverse consequences, *see* problem/s
affective problems 75, 77, 78
Africa 31
Afro-Caribbean groups 115
age factors 68, 77–9, 105, 134, 136, 141–2, 147
aggregate data 50, 53, 54, 102–4
aggression 25, 46, 92, 94, 200
AIDS 163, 168, 180, 184–6, 194–5, 205, 209
alcohol
  abuse 15, 17, 87–94, 151–60, 200
  availability 8, 50–1, 171, 174–6, 184
  aversive effects 152, 153, 183
  in classification systems 87
  craving 61, 183
  and crime 7, 194
  dehydrogenase 151, 152, 153
  dependence syndrome 9, 61, 63, 74, 87, 89, 91, 104
  distilled 17, 20, 22–3, 26–7, 30
  harmful use 89, 92–5
  history of 1–13, 17
  metabolism 151–5, 157
  misuse 15, 17, 29, 99–101
  mode of presentation 70
  and musicians 118
  perceptions of 23, 28, 89, 161, 207
  pharmacological effects 46–7, 94
  policy 22, 54, 167–77, 205–10
  price of 171–4
  pure 18–19, 30
  reinforcing effect of 66
  tolerance of 85, 91, 112
  toxicity 151–60

  see also addiction; consumption; dependence; drinking; problem/s; prohibition
Alcoholics Anonymous 7–8, 17–20, 28–32, 173
alcoholism
  as addiction 7, 180
  classification systems 86–7, 91, 94
  dimensionality 74
  as disease 4–5, 8–9, 28, 30, 61, 85–6, 92, 94, 180
  and genetic factors 152, 153
  Jellinek's species 8, 68–9, 85–6
  prevention of 172
  see also drunkenness; inebriety; intoxication; dependence
Alcohol Problems Questionnaire 74–7
Alcohol Use Inventory 74
America 84, 202–3
  consumption 18, 20, 104–5, 174
  culture 28, 32, 111
  disease concept 5, 28
  drug misuse 114–16, 119, 123
  Epidemiologic Catchment Area Project 136–47
  ethnic groups 111, 113, 154
  prohibition 7, 8, 22, 28, 190
  temperance 15, 16, 23, 27–32
  treatment strategies 184
American Psychiatric Association 84, 89, 91
amphetamines 87, 114, 124, 126
anthropology 110
antidepressants 87, 181
antioxidants 156, 157, 158
anxiety 46, 64, 161–2, 195, 205
Asia and Asians 31, 154
attitudes 94, 119, 122, 167, 174
Australia 16, 19, 20, 27, 29, 31
Austria 19, 21, 30, 31
availability 8, 50–1, 171, 174–6, 184
aversion 152, 153, 183

barbiturates 70, 87, 114, 161–3, 201
Becker, Howard 119–23

Index

beer 18–19, 24, 25, 30
behaviour 85, 91, 92, 95, 174
  causes of 53, 54, 56, 58, 102
  childhood 137, 144–5, 147, 148
  cognitive interventions 184
  destructive 46
  drink-seeking 61
  learned 4, 9
  problematic 86, 100, 107, 200
  research 45
  sexual 46, 94
  and society 64, 69, 71, 79, 145
  see also aggression; delinquency; violence
Belgium 16, 19, 30
benzodiazepines 1–2, 161–6, 201
bi-axial concept 62, 63, 70, 72, 79
biochemistry 206–7
biological factors, *see* genetic factors
biology 193, 199
  psychobiology 63, 64, 95
brain damage 64, 71, 194

Canada 16, 18, 20, 27, 29, 31, 169
cannabis 118–24, 126, 170–75
  in ICD 87
  in India 110–11
  and law 99
  and multiple abuse 145–6
  Wootton Report 209
  and young children 167
Caribbean countries 31, 118, 119
Catholics 21, 24–7, 30, 31
causality 37–59, 66–8, 101–2
  and blame 204
  and different perspectives 179–80, 207
  ecological approach to 103
  and effect 145
  individual vs. culture 133–4
  and statistics 72, 192–3
  theories of 37, 41, 48–9, 52, 58, 73
chaos theory 38, 53, 55
chasing the dragon 114
Cherrington, E.H. 17, 22
children 94, 167, 170
  Adult Children of Alcoholics 15, 28–9, 32
  behaviour of 137, 144–5, 147, 148
  and parents 15, 49–50, 137, 140, 147
cigarettes, *see* smoking
cirrhosis 64, 68, 89, 92, 168, 180, 200
  frequency of 103, 151
  mortality from 50, 72, 173
  predisposition to 94, 152–5, 169, 194
  surgery for 181
  and vitamin deficiency 49

and wine drinkers 26
and Yale Centre for Alcohol Studies 7
classification 5, 63, 83–97, 208
cocaine 94, 126, 145, 170–4, 183, 194
  in classification systems 85, 87
  in nineteenth century 111
community issues 9, 175–6, 191, 202; *see also* culture; social factors
conceptual issues 10
  bi-axial 62, 63, 70, 72, 79
  dependence 61–3, 92, 95
  misuse 99–101
  problem/s 8, 61–3, 95, 101, 161, 179, 199–210
  see also disease concept
constant conjunction 38–41, 58
consumption (of alcohol)
  and abuse 151, 157
  levels of 6, 10, 18–21, 30, 173, 209
  and problems/dependence 61, 70–9, 103–6, 151, 172, 179–80, 186, 191
control
  of availability 8, 171–4, 176, 184
  loss of 7, 24–7, 46, 61, 85
  statistical 49–50, 58
correlations 37–59, 72–3, 134–7, 147
counterfactual analysis 41–5
crack 119, 168, 203
crime 145
  and alcohol 7, 194
  and drugs 112, 116, 202–3
  police arrest 75–8, 95, 101–2, 168, 171
cross-cultural studies 16, 69, 113, 190
cross-sectional methods 72–3, 192
cross-substance comparisons 191
Crothers, T. D. 6, 7, 8
culture/s 68–9, 109–32, 157, 192, 208
  American 28, 32, 111
  cross-cultural studies 16, 69, 95, 113, 190
  development in 54, 58
  drinking 21, 32, 25, 27, 57
  drug 109, 110, 112–13, 203
  English-speaking 15–36
  expectations of 71, 79, 94
  vs. individual factors 133–5, 140–7, 192, 206
  myths 46
  Nordic 15–36
  relativity 100, 110–13, 119
  stereotypes 68–9
  subcultures 110, 113–19, 121–7, 133–4, 148
  temperance 15–36
  see also racial factors; religion; social factors

cure vs. palliation 180-4
cyclizine 114
Czechoslovakia 18, 30

definitions 83, 86, 92
  of addiction 1, 4, 61, 85-7, 92, 161, 179
  of alcoholism 95
  of causality 37, 38
  of culture 109-10
  of dependence 87
  of drug misuse 110
  of problem/s 100, 161-6, 167, 190-1, 199-210
  see also conceptual issues
dehydrogenase 151, 152, 153
delinquency 116, 144, 145, 148
delusional symptoms 92
Denmark 18, 20, 21, 27, 30
dependence 5, 140, 202
  benzodiazepines 164-5, 194
  in classification systems 87, 91-5
  concept of 61-3, 92, 95
  and consumption 61, 70-9, 103-6, 151, 172, 179-80, 186, 191
  and disease 9, 30, 61, 167, 179
  levels of 74-7, 106, 168-9
  normal dose 2, 164
  pharmacological 92, 117
  and prevention 167, 172-3
  and problem/s 1-13, 61-82, 85, 92, 101, 164-5, 172, 186, 200
  syndrome 9, 61, 63, 74, 87, 89, 91, 104
  tobacco 171
  withdrawal symptoms
depression 64, 75, 89, 92, 146-7, 181, 195
designer drugs 194
determinism 38, 53-7
deviance 112, 116, 144
diagnostic systems 63, 83-4, 89-95
dimensionality 9, 10, 208
dipsomania 4, 5, 84, 85, 86
disabilities 1, 8, 86, 89, 179; *see also* problem/s
disease concept 2-10, 85-6, 92-5, 179-80
  and dependence 9, 30, 61, 167, 179
  and temperance 5-6, 26, 28, 85
distilled liquor 17, 20, 22-3, 26-7, 30
doctors 3, 5-6, 61, 117-19, 165, 201
dose 2, 161-4, 204
drink, *see* alcohol
drinking 6, 7, 9,
  careers 52, 54, 67
  controlled 184
  culture 57
  excessive 86, 87

moderate 30
  patterns 20, 23, 71, 79, 151
  public concern about 28, 61
  safe levels of 171
  social 171
  style 105, 106
  see also alcohol
driving 28-9, 32, 64-5, 94, 169-70
drug/s
  abuse 87, 89, 93, 163-4, 173
  availability 174, 176, 184
  and creativity 117-18
  criminalization of 112
  and culture 109-32, 203
  designer 194
  experiences of 125-8
  experimentation 120
  formulation of 114, 162, 163
  illegal 171-4, 191, 194-5, 202, 205
  injection 113-16, 163-4, 184, 195, 209
  method of administration 70, 114
  nosology of problems 85, 87
  perceptions of 28, 89, 122, 161, 207
  pharmacological effects 109, 110, 113, 117, 120, 124-5
  regulation of 112
  snorting 114
  substitution 184
  tourism 112
  trafficking 99, 174
  see also addiction; dependence; problem/s
drunkenness 1, 2-5, 6, 15, 20-3, 84, 87;
  see also alcoholism
Durkheim, Emile 24-6, 31, 55

economic factors 6, 16, 68, 77, 104, 208
education 115, 116, 173-6, 184
eighteenth century 2, 3, 70, 110
emotional problems 144-5
empirical methods 38-41, 44, 63, 72, 79-80, 193
employment 6, 102, 106, 116-19, 168, 204
environmental factors, *see* culture
Epidemiologic Catchment Area Project 136-47
epidemiology 9, 102, 104, 185
epistemology 37-59
ethanol, *see* alcohol
ethnic groups, *see* racial factors
experimental methods 9, 37, 44-8, 50, 52, 58

facial flushing 152, 153, 154
family 6, 28, 100, 168, 194
  substance abuse in 136-7, 140, 148
fetal damage 194

Finland 15–16, 18, 20, 28–9, 31
flushing 152, 153, 154
formulation of drugs 114, 162, 163
France 10, 16, 19, 21, 26, 30, 85, 94
free radicals 151, 156, 157, 158
friendship networks 115, 146

gender factors 68, 134, 136
  alcohol use 77–9, 104, 151, 153, 169
  drug use 113–16, 119
  Epidemiologic Catchment Area Project 140–1, 147
genetic factors 5, 137, 179, 193–4, 207–8
  vs. environment 140, 157
  ethnic variation 152–4
Germany 19–24, 30, 31, 85, 112
gin 17, 22
Greece 21

habit 2–5, 9, 119–22, 191; *see also* addiction; dependence
hallucinogens 87, 123
hard liquor 17, 20, 22–3, 26–7, 30
harmful use of alcohol 89, 92–5
harm-reduction interventions 115, 182–4, 186
health economics 6, 193
health education 115, 116, 173–6, 184
health promotion 175
heart disease 155, 175, 181
heavy use 137–48, 168, 172, 173
hepatic cirrhosis, *see* cirrhosis
heroin 26, 113–10, 122–8, 144–6, 180, 183, 186
hippie subculture 121–4
history 1–13, 17, 84–6, 190, 199, 207
HIV infection 163, 168, 180, 184–6, 194–5, 205, 209
Holland 20, 30
homeorhesis 54, 55
Hume, David 37, 38–41, 44, 52
Hungary 19, 30
hypnotics 161, 163, 164
  see also benzodiazepines; barbiturates

Iceland 16, 18, 20
illegal drugs 171–4, 191, 194–5, 202, 205
indeterminism 53, 54, 55, 58
India and Indians 110–11, 154
individual/s 133–60
  and prevention policy 167, 206
  problem research 193–4
  self-control 24–7
  in social context 69, 99–108, 192

inebriety 4, 5, 61, 85, 87; *see also* alcoholism
injection 113–16, 163–4, 184, 195, 209
  see also harm reduction
insomnia 92, 162
international classification systems 83–97
intoxicants 2, 110, 111
intoxication 85, 87, 91, 92, 95; *see also* alcoholism
Ireland 18, 21, 30
Islamic societies 2, 69, 94
Italy 16, 19, 21, 25–6, 30

Jellinek, E. M. 4, 7–8, 10, 68–9, 85–6, 168
Jews 24, 142
job loss 116–17, 168, 204

Kerr, N. 6, 7, 8
Kraepelin, Emil 85, 89

language 125–8
law 99, 111, 112, 171, 184
  of large numbers 55–6
learning 4, 9, 95, 119, 120
life events 68, 137, 146, 147
lifestyles 110, 116, 117, 119, 205
liver cirrhosis, *see* cirrhosis
loss of control 7, 24–7, 46, 61, 85
LSD 120, 121–8

macro-level phenomena 53, 55, 56
mania 146, 147
marijuana, *see* cannabis
marital problems 66–7, 102, 145, 168
mass media 169, 173, 175
mathematics 10, 52, 56
medical profession 3, 5–6, 61, 117–19, 165, 201
medicine 3, 10, 83, 85, 199, 210
men 21, 28, 115, 134, 140–3, 151
  prevention policies 169, 175
mental health/illness 61, 64, 133, 137, 145–8, 179
  in classification systems 84–5
  and life events 68
  see also psychiatry
meprobamate 163
metabolism of alcohol 151–5, 157
methadone 184
methedrine 124
methodology
  balanced placebo design 46
  cross-cultural studies 16, 69, 113, 190

cross-sectional studies 72–3, 192
experimental 9, 37, 44–8, 50, 52, 58
life events 68, 137, 146, 147
longitudinal studies 192
non-experimental 37–8, 48–53, 58
observational 194
path analysis 2, 4, 73, 78
pluralism of 38, 48
questionnaires 74–7
regression analysis 73, 77, 78, 107
spuriousness 40–1, 43–5, 49–50, 58, 73
see also research; science
Mexico 31
Michigan Alcoholism Screening Test (MAST) 172
micro-level phenomena 53, 55, 56
misuse 15, 17, 29, 99–101, 110, 112–19; *see also* abuse
models 91, 101, 104, 107, 179–80
 animal 148
 biological 207
 causal 72
 historical 2, 4, 6, 8
 mathematical 52, 56
 medical/disease 92, 94–5, 147, 167
moral issues 23, 61, 111, 179, 202, 208
morphine 85, 87, 146
mortality 26, 50, 72, 170, 173, 191
 suicide 24, 75, 200, 203–4
musicians 117–19
Muslim societies 2, 69, 94
myopathy 155, 156, 157, 193

naltrexone 183
narcotics 85, 144, 190
neo-temperance 28, 32
Netherlands 18, 21, 30, 112, 119
New Zealand 16, 19, 20
nicotine 5, 184; *see also* smoking
nineteenth century 1, 5, 61, 84–5, 92, 110–11
 temperance movements 15–17, 20–8, 32
nomenclature 83–4, 85–7, 89, 92
non-experimental methods 48–53, 58
Norway 16, 18, 20, 26, 30, 49, 51–2, 200
nutrition factors 68, 158

occupation 6, 116–19, 168, 204
opiates 125–6, 181, 183, 194, 202, 208
 in classification systems 85
 and multidrug abuse 145
 in nineteenth century 111
opium 1, 5, 110, 111, 190
overdose 161, 162, 204

palliation vs. cure 180–4
pancreatitis 94, 194
parasuicide 161, 162, 204
parents 15, 49–50, 137, 140, 147
path analysis 2, 4, 73, 78
patterns of use and misuse 20, 23, 71, 79, 113–15, 151
peer groups 148, 174
peptic ulcers 181
perceptions 23, 28, 89, 122, 161, 207
personality factors 68, 91, 94, 145–6, 148, 179
pharmaceutical industry 165
pharmacology 193
 of dependence 92, 117
 vs. other effects 46–7, 94, 109–10, 113, 119–26
psychopharmacology 119, 120, 124, 199
phenycyclidine 94
philosophy 37, 44, 199, 208
physical problems 61, 64, 75, 77, 168, 208
 and barbiturates 70
 cause of 102
 in classification systems 85, 89, 92
physics 207–8
physiology 8
Poland 18, 20, 23, 30, 32
police, *see* crime
policy issues 22, 54, 167–77, 205, 207, 209–10
political factors 16, 22, 204
polydrug abuse 145, 163
population/s
 clinical 65, 79, 183, 191
 community 9, 175–6, 191, 202
 vs. individuals 99
 research 191–3
 target 147, 169–70, 173, 176
Portugal 19, 21, 30
poverty 6, 116, 203
predictability 38–9, 54, 63, 79, 103
predisposition, *see* genetic factors; vulnerability
pregnant women 32, 116
prescribing 162, 165
prevalence of problems 6, 9
prevention 8, 167–77, 206
price control 171–4, 184
problem/s 6, 69
 adverse effects 162–3, 201
 affective 75, 77, 78
 and classification systems 83–97
 concept of 8, 61–3, 95, 101, 161, 179, 199–210
 and consumption 61, 70–9, 103–6, 151, 172, 179–80, 186, 191

definition of 100, 161–6, 167, 190–1, 199–210
and dependence 1–13, 61–82, 85, 92, 101, 164–5, 172, 186, 200
emotional 144–5
epistemological 37–59
extensive use 161–2
financial 21, 75, 77, 78
friendship 75, 77
levels of 168–9
marital 66–7, 102, 145, 168
measurement of 63
ontological 45
organic, *see* physical problems
police, *see* crime
prevalence of 6, 9
and prevention policies 167–77
progression of 135, 145–6
psychiatric, *see* mental health/illness
psychological 75–7, 85–6, 89, 92, 95, 194, 208
research 189–97
social, *see* social problems
in temperance cultures 15–36
and treatment strategies 179–88
see also abuse; addiction; behaviour; employment; family; misuse; poverty
prohibition 7, 8, 22, 28, 190
prostitutes 117–19
Protestants 17, 20, 21, 24–7, 30–2
psychedelics 123, 124
psychiatry 5, 83, 85, 89–91, 199, 208; *see also* mental health/illness
psychoactive substances 61, 83, 148, 201–2, 206
in classification systems 87, 92
and religion 142
psychobiology 63, 64, 95
psychological problems 75–7, 85–6, 89, 92, 95, 194, 208; *see also* mental health/illness
psychology 5, 46–7, 85, 193, 206
psychopathology 84, 164
psychopharmacology 119, 120, 124, 199
psychoses 85, 120, 123, 146
psychosurgery 183
psychotherapy 183
public health 5, 6, 7, 8, 83, 203

quantum mechanics 53, 54, 57, 58
questionnaires 74–7

racial factors 113–16, 137, 140–4, 147, 151–4, 201
real-life situations 48, 51, 54, 107

regression analysis 73, 77, 78, 107
religion 24, 111, 142, 208
see also Catholics; Islamic societies; Jews; Protestants
research 9, 189–97
clinical 63, 65, 74, 79
empirical 38–41, 44, 63, 72, 79–80, 193
epistemological problems 37–59
multidisciplinary 193, 194, 196, 206
prevention 176
problem-orientated 189–97
qualitative and quantitative 194
statistics 49–50, 58, 63, 72–9, 107, 192–3
survey 65, 73, 107, 191–3
treatment 47–8, 74
see also methodology; science
risk-taking 115, 116
Roman Catholics 21, 24–7, 30, 31
Romania 21
rum 17, 22
Rush, Benjamin 3, 4, 5, 61, 70, 84–5
Russia 17, 18, 20–3, 30, 94

safe levels of drinking 171
Scandinavia 10, 15–36
schizophrenia 146, 147
science 10, 63, 200–10
social 10, 206
see also methodology; research
Scotland 114
sedatives 116, 145, 164
self-control 24–7
self-help approaches 15, 173, 184
set and setting 46, 120, 122–5
Severity of Alcohol Dependence Questionnaire 74–7
sex, *see* gender factors
sexual behaviour 46, 94
sharing syringes 113–16
sinfulness 2, 3
smoking 87, 111–16, 171–2, 174, 186, 190–1, 208
snorting drugs 114
social anthropology 110
social drinking and drug use 171
social factors 48, 55–7, 94, 111, 201–3
class 77, 78, 79, 104–6
deprivation 116, 179, 203–4
disapproval 71, 79
networks 68, 100, 115, 146
norms 69, 71, 79, 94
socialization 110, 115–16, 119–22, 134
social problems 15, 21, 23, 61, 168, 208
in classification systems 85–6, 92–5

and drug cultures 203
and individual behaviour 69, 194
social science 10, 206
sociology 17, 193, 199, 203, 206
Soviet Union 17, 18, 20–3, 30, 94
Spain 19, 21, 30
spirits 18–21, 22–4, 25–7, 30
spuriousness 40–1, 43–5, 49–50, 58, 73
Stanford Heart Disease Prevention Project 175
statistics 49–50, 58, 63, 72–9, 107, 192–3
　see also methodology
stereotypes 68–9
stimulants 118, 145
strokes 170
subcultures 110, 113–19, 121–7, 133–4, 148
substance/s 1, 114
　abuse 37–59, 91, 94–5, 133–50, 161
　levels of use 133, 208
　psychoactive 61, 83, 87, 92, 201, 206
　use disorders 84, 85, 88, 90–2, 95
　see also addiction; alcohol; dependence; drug/s; problem/s
suicide 24, 75, 200, 203–4
Suppes, P. 37, 48–9, 73
survey research 65, 73, 107, 191–3
Sweden 16, 18, 20, 26–7, 30–1, 51, 141, 172
Switzerland 19, 20, 21, 24, 30, 31, 112

taxation 184, 209
temazepam 114, 163
temperance 5–6, 15–36, 61, 85
theories 61, 70–2, 107, 193
　action 44, 58
　of causality 37, 41, 48–9, 52, 58, 73
　chaos 38, 53, 55
　and empirical findings 79–80, 193
　labelling 112, 190
　social reaction 112
time factors 64–6, 72–3, 170
tissues 151, 155–7, 194
tobacco, *see* smoking
tolerance 85, 91, 112, 165
toxicity 151–60, 162
trafficking 99, 174
tranquillizers 87, 114, 116, 145, 162–4
treatment 29–30, 48, 63, 179–88
　campaigns 5, 6, 8
　research 47–8, 74
　services 115, 173
Trotter, Thomas 3, 4, 5, 181
Troubles With Drinking Questionnaire 74

twentieth century 4, 6–8, 92, 111
　temperance movements 15–17, 21, 24, 26–8, 30

Ukraine 17
Ulster 21
unemployment 116–17, 168, 204
United States, *see* America
unpredictability 39, 54
use 133, 161–2, 201–3, 208
　disorders 84, 85, 88, 90–2, 95
　harmful 89, 92–5
　heavy 137–48, 168, 172, 173
　patterns 20, 23, 71, 79, 113–15, 151
　social 171
　see also abuse; consumption; misuse

validity 48, 51, 52, 53
valium 162
variables 52, 77–8, 104–7
　cultural vs. individual 134–7, 147–8, 192
　intervening 73, 75
Vietnam veterans 141, 146, 147
violence 25, 163, 168, 169, 194
vitamins 49, 151, 156, 157, 206
vodka 17, 22, 23
vulnerability factors 68, 77–9, 151–60
　to alcohol addiction 8, 95
　cultural and individual 94, 116, 133, 147–8, 208

Weber, Max 24–6, 31
whiskey 17, 22
Willis, Paul 121–2
wine 18–19, 21, 24–6, 30, 32
withdrawal symptoms 61, 75, 77, 85–6, 91, 164–5
women 21, 28, 78, 140, 142–3, 201
　alcohol metabolism 151–5
　benzodiazepine use 162
　pregnant 32, 116
　preventive policy for 169, 173, 175
　socialization of 115–16, 134
work 6, 102, 106, 116–19, 168, 204
World Health Organization 1, 7–10, 30, 62, 99, 204
　and classification systems 86, 87, 89

young people 109–10, 116, 141, 168–70, 173–4, 201, 205
Yugoslavia 17